'One of the most surprising things about yoga is that it's primarily concerned with working with the mind. Yet most yoga teachers have very little training around mental health and how yoga might impact us both emotionally and mentally. In *Mental Health Aware Yoga*, Dr Lauren Tober offers an integration of Eastern wisdom and Western psychology and shares a practical approach to support our mental health and the mental health of our students. This is essential reading for yoga teachers and yoga therapists since almost half of our students will experience a diagnosed mental health condition in their lifetime.'

– Jivana Heyman, director of Accessible Yoga

'*Mental Health Aware Yoga* offers teachers the knowledge and confidence to identify psycho-emotional states and guidelines for meeting the students "where they are" with appropriate practices that lead toward balance, self-regulation and, in yogic terms, a sattvic state. You will find practice gems to meet and manage mood and, equally important, you'll understand what practices and language to avoid. If you teach yoga, this book belongs on your bookshelf!'

– Amy Weintraub, author of *Yoga for Depression*, *Yoga Skills for Therapists* and the *Yoga For Your Mood Deck*

'*Mental Health Aware Yoga* is a beacon of light, masterfully guiding yoga practitioners and teachers through the intertwined paths of mental wellness and yoga with warmth and wisdom. Lauren's deep expertise shines in her practical approach to the six pillars of Mental Health Aware Yoga, rooted in decades of clinical and personal experience. This book is an invitation to a community of growth, and a testament to the power of yoga as a tool for healing. Join Lauren's transformative dialogue and become part of a movement towards holistic health and compassionate teaching.'

– Richard Miller, PhD, founder and director of the iRest Center and developer of Integr[illegible] on iRest Meditation, [illegible]w.iRestCenter.com

'*Mental Health Aware Yoga* is a groundbreaking book that every yoga teacher needs to read, whether they are just starting out on their teaching journey or have been teaching for decades. With so many people turning to yoga for mental health reasons these days, it is essential that yoga teachers have solid mental health knowledge. This easy-to-digest book will help you to support your students compassionately and confidently and will change the way you teach yoga. *Mental Health Aware Yoga* is destined to become a classic and a staple in all yoga teacher training courses!'

– Stephen Cope, bestselling author of *Yoga and the Quest for the True Self* and scholar in residence at the Kripalu Center for Yoga and Health

'The book is an easy read with everything you want to know on the subject, well-referenced and presented in a lucid manner. I especially found the pointers to look for in a classroom relating to different conditions and the compassionate reflection guide interesting and useful. I highly recommend this book for all serious yoga teachers who want to make yoga accessible and most beneficial for themselves and their students.'

– Saraswathi Vasudevan, co-founder of Yoga Vahini

'Lauren Tober's *Mental Health Aware Yoga* is a vibrant exploration into the healing power of yoga through a somatic lens. It's a compelling invitation to deepen our understanding of the body-mind connection and a truly powerful tool for mental, emotional and physical wellbeing.'

– Dr Scott Lyons, founder of The Embody Lab

Mental Health Aware Yoga

of related interest

Yoga for Mental Health
Edited by Heather Mason and Kelly Birch
Forewords by B. N. Gangadhar and Timothy McCall
ISBN 978 1 90914 135 3
eISBN 978 1 91208 526 2

Trauma-Informed and Trauma-Responsive Yoga Teaching
A Universal Practice
Catherine Cook-Cottone and Joanne Spence
Forewords by Dr. Shirley Telles and Dr. Gail Parker
ISBN 978 1 83997 816 6
eISBN 978 1 83997 817 3

Yin Yoga Therapy and Mental Health
An Integrated Approach
Tracey Meyers, Psy.D.
Foreword by Sarah Powers
ISBN 978 1 84819 415 1
eISBN 978 0 85701 383 5

Yoga Therapy for Stress, Burnout and Chronic Fatigue Syndrome
Fiona Agombar
Foreword by Alex Howard
Contributions by Leah Barnett
ISBN 978 1 84819 277 5
eISBN 978 0 85701 223 4

The Science of Movement, Exercise, and Mental Health
Jennifer Pilotti
ISBN 978 1 83997 773 2
eISBN 978 1 83997 774 9

MENTAL HEALTH AWARE YOGA

A Guide for Yoga Teachers

Dr Lauren Tober

SINGING DRAGON
LONDON AND PHILADELPHIA

First published in Great Britain in 2024 by Singing Dragon,
an imprint of Jessica Kingsley Publishers
Part of John Murray Press

3

A CIP catalogue record for this title is available from the
British Library and the Library of Congress

ISBN 978 1 80501 227 6
eISBN 978 1 80501 228 3

Printed and bound by CPI Group (UK) Ltd, Croydon, CR0 4YY

Jessica Kingsley Publishers' policy is to use papers that are natural, renewable and recyclable products and made from wood grown in sustainable forests. The logging and manufacturing processes are expected to conform to the environmental regulations of the country of origin.

Singing Dragon
Carmelite House
50 Victoria Embankment
London EC4Y 0DZ

www.singingdragon.com

John Murray Press
Part of Hodder & Stoughton Limited
An Hachette UK Company

Disclaimer

The information provided in this book is intended to be for informational purposes only and does not constitute or replace professional individualized psychological advice or yoga training. While the author is a clinical psychologist and yoga teacher, this book is not a psychological service nor a yoga teacher training program.

For individualized mental health support, please see a health care provider, and for yoga teachers seeking mental health training, please consider joining the Mental Health Aware Yoga training at www.mentalhealthawareyoga.com.

Dr Lauren Tober

Yoga Psychology Institute

Bundjalung country, Mullumbimby, Australia

www.mentalhealthawareyoga.com

For Lukas, who reminded me that books always need a dedication and he would be the best person to dedicate it to. And for Zaia, who, at age 11, has been writing her first book at the same time that I have been writing mine.

I love you both more than I know how to put into words.

Contents

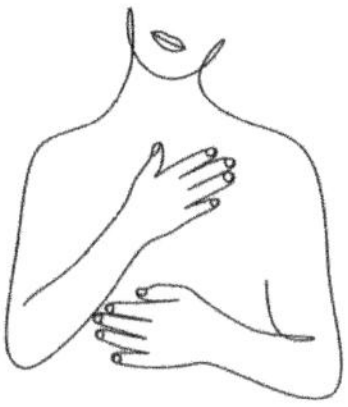

INTRODUCTION

ABOUT THIS BOOK

Thank you for picking up this book. The very fact that you have shows me that you are someone who cares deeply about the mental health and happiness of the world, your students, and (hopefully) yourself.

And we need more people, and more yoga teachers like you in the world.

We may not be sitting together in the same room having these conversations about yoga and mental health, but know that as I am writing this, that is exactly what I am imagining. In my mind, we are sitting together on cushions and yoga bolsters, sharing a pot of tea, and having conversations about yoga, mental health, connection, happiness, healing, growth, inclusivity, community and surviving and thriving in the face of adversity.

So pull up a cushion, light a candle, pour yourself a cuppa and let us dive in.

This book has evolved from the Mental Health Aware Yoga training program, a professional development training course that educates and inspires yoga teachers to support their students experiencing depression, anxiety, stress and trauma.

In this book, just like in the training, we will explore the six pillars of Mental Health Aware Yoga, including:

1. Western Psychology

2. Yoga Psychology

3. Safe Container
4. Therapeutic Skills
5. Yogic Practices
6. Mental Health Crisis.

By the end of this book, my hope is that you will have a clear understanding of the role that yoga can play in overcoming mental health challenges and fostering positive mental health and have started to bring some of these ideas into your teaching and into your life. I have also provided additional resources online to support your ongoing learning and development at www.mentalhealthawareyoga.com/book-resources. I would love to share these with you, so do go and download them right away!

This book draws on over two decades of my clinical, teaching and personal experience, as well as drawing largely on the work of many great teachers, researchers, authors and scholars. While at times it may seem cumbersome, I have attempted to reference all these sources, including translations and interpretations of yogic texts and more recent scientific research and commentaries. As I am not a yogic scholar myself, my understanding of the yogic texts I have shared comes from a number of interpretations, both written and oral, particularly Saraswathi Vasudevan, T.K.V. Desikachar, Edwin F. Bryant, Susanna Barkataki, Anand Mehotra and Richard Miller, and hence I have referenced them consistently throughout. For consistency, throughout this manual I have used the Sanskrit notations from T.K.V. Desikachar's *The Heart of Yoga*, except where I have quoted another source, and in that instance I have directly quoted their notations.

I am deeply grateful for my yoga teachers (and there have been many over the years) and their teachers, and their teachers before them, and all those sharing the wisdom of yoga, from teacher to student for thousands of years.

This work is constantly evolving, both as the collective understanding of these topics evolve, but also as my own personal understanding of it unfolds and matures. I bow in deep gratitude to all those who have come before me and those who have shone a light on my own ignorance and blind spots, and I humbly ask for grace as I continue to navigate these, and take the bold step of publishing a book knowing that what I share today will likely become refined or outdated tomorrow. I wish this for us all! That we show up in the world as our whole selves, with depth, authenticity and humbleness, and continue to grow and refine what we believe to be true.

This book is simply the beginning. I hope it will introduce you to some of the important principles of Mental Health Aware Yoga, and inspire you to use this knowledge to support your students experiencing mental health challenges. If this work resonates with you, I invite you to join us for the Mental Health Aware Yoga training and join our worldwide directory of Mental Health Aware Yoga Teachers. You can find out more at www.mentalhealthawareyoga.com.

Thank you for taking this first step with me.

A NOTE ON TAKING CARE OF YOURSELF

Conversations about mental health are not always easy, particularly if you have your own lived experience of mental health challenges, or love someone who has.

But they are important. And I am so glad you are here.

If you feel uncomfortable, overwhelmed or triggered at any time while you are reading this book, then the invitation is to pause, put down the book and do whatever you need to do to feel okay again. This might be one of the yoga practices you will read about in the Yogic Practices chapter, but it also might be hugging someone you love, going outside and putting your bare feet on the earth, walking in nature, turning up the music and dancing it out or using it as an opportunity for further self-enquiry and healing through journalling, meditation or by bringing it to your next therapy session.

I know as yoga teachers we sometimes think that we need to have it all together all of the time, but the reality is that we are human, and we all go through challenging times and need support too.

So please take care of yourself, bring a big dose of self-compassion to this work and reach out to your support team of friends, family, mentors and therapists whenever you need.

We are all in this together.

MY STORY

I started yoga at 21, in a community centre in downtown Vancouver.

I had arrived as an exchange student at the University of British Columbia, and had found myself transported, just days before Christmas and while nursing a broken heart, from sunny Australia to icy cold Canada. I did not know a single person. After spending Christmas Day alone, watching old Beatles movies at the cinema and eating poutine for the first (and last) time, I was befriended by a guy who worked at the youth hostel I was staying at.

He introduced me to homemade brownies and Kundalini Yoga. Both made my head spin.

We attended my very first yoga class at the downtown community centre, in a dark room at the top of many flights of stairs, lit only by fairy lights. The large room was packed with people from all walks of life, and the teachers were dressed in all white, complete with white fabric wrapped around their heads. We did what I now know was some pretty extreme prāṇāyāma and āsana practices, and chanted *may the long-time sun shine upon you*. To say it was outside my comfort zone would be an understatement.

I grew up in a country town in Australia, in a pretty conservative middle-class community in a time before yoga was part of popular culture, and so it all looked and felt suspiciously like a cult to me. Exactly the kind of thing that my parents would have been concerned about if they knew what I was doing. Quite possibly that was part of the attraction!

If I am honest, I did not really enjoy that first class. It was physically challenging and felt very strange. But I did have a sense that it was going to change my life and I needed to keep doing it.

So I did.

And as I was studying psychology, sexuality and the philosophy of science at the University of British Columbia, I went to yoga classes whenever I could. Fortuitously, I ended up as a nanny for a young boy whose mother had a house full of books on yoga and meditation, and I devoured everything I could on the topic.

By the time I had finished the semester and headed off backpacking around Europe, I was well and truly down the yogic rabbit hole, so to speak. But while I had a sporadic yoga āsana practice and had taken the first yama, ahiṁsā, to heart by becoming vegetarian, my knowledge of yoga was mostly academic, from what I had gleaned from books in my boss' house and bought in secondhand bookshops.

It took me many years to bring yoga and meditation off the page and out of my head, and to become an embodied part of my life.

A few years later

After finishing my psychology studies and internship back in Australia, I qualified and registered as a psychologist, and did what many young Australians do: I headed to London with a working holiday visa and moved into a massive dilapidated share house full of foreigners.

Previously, I had been lucky enough to have been offered a coveted psychology internship in community and mental health, and accepted it, mostly because when I looked around at all the other graduate jobs on offer there was not a single job I could imagine myself doing. Even then I knew I was not cut out for a corporate or bureaucratic career, even though everyone around me was headed in that direction. A friend told me that I had *delusions of grandeur* for wanting something different. But after the two-year internship program, at the ripe old age of 24, I felt completely underprepared and lacked confidence in my ability to help anyone.

Hence, London.

England did not recognize my Australian psychology qualifications, and I was not sure I wanted to be a psychologist anyway, so I took a job helping *underprivileged* kids find work. I earned £9 an hour in one of the most expensive cities in the world, doing a job that was demoralizing, both for the young people I worked with and myself. There were no jobs for these young people, no matter how hard I tried.

But the gold that came out of my time in London was an apprenticeship in Ashtanga Yoga. In my twenties, Ashtanga was just what I needed to harness my busy mind and, if I am honest, the demanding physical practice probably fed my ego too. So, a few times a week I trekked across the city on the tube and trained to become an Ashtanga Yoga teacher.

The apprenticeship was very hands-on, both in terms of the Ashtanga-style adjustments I was taught to provide and also in terms of the practical nature of the apprenticeship. There was no reading of any yogic texts or material, and instead I was given an on-the-job crash course in teaching yoga. I guess it fitted with Pattabhi Jois' often touted claim of '99% practice, 1% theory'.

The classes I assisted in were taught in a beautiful old building, in a large room on the first floor, with high ceilings and wooden floorboards. The *beginner* students were led through a variation of the primary series in the back of the room, and the more *advanced* students practised *Mysore Style*, moving through the sequence at their own pace with the teacher offering one-on-one support and hands-on adjustments at the front of the room.

I observed and assisted the senior teachers for some time before I was thrown into the deep end and given the beginner's class to teach. While I had taught contemporary dance classes and a few kids yoga classes before, it was my first time teaching yoga to adults, and I remember vividly how terrified I was to lead that first chant and teach an entire yoga class to a group of earnest students. The relief I felt when the students reached Śavāsana at the end of the primary series was palpable.

And, to be fair, the relief was probably felt by the students too. Ashtanga Yoga is a pretty physically demanding practice!

Home to India

When the apprenticeship ended, and with very little holding me in London, my boyfriend (now husband) and I made our way overland from Germany to Iran, and then flew across the border to study yoga in India.

I immediately felt like I had come home.

While I had grown up on stories of my parents backpacking around India and other parts of the world in the 1970s, I had never been there myself. It was busy, noisy and intense, people stared at us all the time, it smelled like nothing I had ever smelled before and yet it felt like home.

I spent the good part of a year studying classical and Ashtanga Yoga in Bengaluru and Mysuru, and felt the freedom of having nothing else to do but study yoga, eat dosas, read books and ride around the countryside on a motorbike. That may have been one of the freest times of my life!

I learned so much about practising and teaching yoga in India, but one of the biggest lessons was that gurus are fallible people too, just like the rest of us. I went to India with an idea of finding a teacher or guru to enlighten me about the meaning of life, but after seeing the human-ness of the men I was studying with, I dropped this idea pretty quickly. I now believe that the sooner we stop looking for someone to put on a pedestal and hand over our life decisions to, the better off we are all going to be. And the abuse and inappropriate behaviour I have seen in the years since have only reinforced this.

While I loved India and loved studying yoga there, I was left feeling pretty baffled about what yoga actually was. My Western academic mind wanted bullet points and executive summaries, and instead our philosophy classes started with 'yes, please?' and a head wiggle, which I think meant 'what would you like to learn today?' As far as I could discern, much of the time, there was no syllabus. Just a willingness to talk about whatever topic was relevant on the day.

Years later, I tried bringing elements of this approach into one of the yoga teacher trainings I was teaching on in Australia. I wanted to honour my Indian teachers and at the same time try to meet the needs of my Australian students by offering both the bullet points *and* the more go-with-the-flow approach I had experienced in India. I am not sure why I was surprised when it did not go down so well, and some of the students gave some pretty negative feedback to the course co-ordinator afterwards! Australian minds seem to like structure and categorization, and we all seem to get a little lost without it.

This is part of the reason that I have introduced the six pillars of Mental Health Aware Yoga in this book and the Mental Health Aware Yoga training. I have learned how important it is to *meet your students where they are* and, for most of us in the Western world, the need for structure is where we are at. However, if you take the Mental Health Aware Yoga training with me, while you probably will not see me wiggle my head Indian style and ask 'yes, please?', you will see me open up for questions and comments and hear me say 'tell me more about that', which is really just a psychologist's way of wiggling our heads and saying 'yes, please?', without the cultural appropriation.

Towards the end of our stay in India, and after much soul searching, I decided that I wanted to be a psychologist after all, and integrate yoga and mental health in my work. But I also realized how grossly underprepared I was to actually be a psychologist, and how little I knew about yoga for mental health. So, from a shonky internet connection in Mysuru, I applied for a doctorate in clinical psychology at the Australian National University to study yoga and clinical psychology.

My interview to get into this prestigious program at one of Australia's top universities was via phone (this was before video calls reliably worked). The program director called me on the Nokia flip phone I had bought in London, and I had the interview pacing around in a small field across the road from my teacher's yoga shala, trying to get reception, while the rest of the class was learning how to use neti pots, letting the warm salty water drip through their nasal passages onto the road next to where I was standing. The contrast could not have been greater.

Back to the books

Somehow, I was accepted into the doctoral program. With hundreds of applications and fewer than 20 students accepted, I am still not sure how I was offered a place. My undergraduate grades were good, but they were not *that* good. I was always more interested in yoga, travel and photography than I was in exams. I can only imagine that it must have been the interview from the field in India that tipped the scale!

When I arrived back in Australia in 2007, with my mala beads, om necklace and Buddha statues, fresh off the plane from India (I am cringing now as I write this), I was fired up and enthusiastic about writing my doctoral thesis on yoga and mental health.

In my first session with my thesis supervisor, the head of the clinical psychology program, I told him my idea to research a topic related to yoga and mental health, and he looked over at me with his fingers poised above the keyboard ready to search the library journal articles, gave me a quizzical look and asked: 'How do you spell yoga?'

In one short sentence, my dreams came tumbling down.

I had the desire and enthusiasm to research yoga and mental health, but none of the research skills required to take on a three-year doctoral project by myself, without the support of the university.

In the end, we compromised and I focused on mindfulness-based cognitive therapy (MBCT), a well-researched and highly regarded treatment for recurrent depression that integrates cognitive therapy, mindfulness meditation and (although they do not talk about it in academic circles) yoga.

Previously, the research had only looked at individuals with a sole diagnosis of depression but, in reality, depression and anxiety are often co-morbid, meaning that they often occur together. My research found that MBCT was helpful in reducing levels of both depression and anxiety in individuals with co-morbid depression and anxiety.

Byron Bay, the Yoga Capital of Australia

In 2009, at seven months pregnant and halfway through finishing my doctoral thesis, my husband and I moved to the Byron Shire.

It really was not until I moved to this yoga capital of Australia that I felt able to truly begin to bring the fields of yoga and psychology together.

In Canberra, we ran a small Ashtanga Yoga school and I worked as a psychologist, but these two worlds were quite separate. I brought a little mindfulness into my clinical practice, but did not really know how to bring them together in a way that was helpful and acceptable for clients and fitted within the health system I was working in. However, in Byron Bay, I began teaching Yoga for Depression and Yoga for Anxiety courses, integrating what I knew about yoga and mental health.

I loved teaching these classes, and the feedback I had from my students was great, but the more I taught them, the more redundant it felt to teach courses specifically for depression and anxiety. You see, what I was teaching was not really that different from what I would teach in a regular, well-rounded yoga class that was sensitive to the needs of the students. And it had me questioning the need for specific mental health yoga classes.

What if, I wondered, all yoga teachers were mental health aware, and students who were experiencing depression and anxiety could go to a regular yoga class, without the expense or stigma of attending a specialized class?

In theory, this made a lot of sense to me. But when I looked around at the classes on offer, I realized that many yoga teachers really did not understand mental health.

The way I saw it, yoga itself was wonderful for mental health, but the way it was taught was not always conducive to positive mental health. Unfortunately, as you probably know, most yoga teacher trainings just do not include mental health education in the curriculum, so it is no wonder that yoga teachers do not always have a solid understanding of mental health and how yoga can help.

But with nearly 80% of yoga students reporting that they practice yoga for the mental health benefits,[1] it is unbelievably important that yoga teachers understand how to support their students experiencing mental health challenges in their classes.

So, I decided to do something about it, and spent a year creating the Mental Health Aware Yoga training, an in-depth course to teach yoga teachers about mental health, so they could support their students experiencing mental health challenges.

Now do not get me wrong, I still think there is a time and a place for specialist classes for mental health. But I wholeheartedly believe that regular yoga classes with a Mental Health Aware Yoga teacher is just as good, if not better at times, than specialized classes. There is no stigma, they are more readily available and often more affordable and accessible.

I taught the Mental Health Aware Yoga training here in Australia and in Europe in 2019 and early 2020, and when COVID turned the world upside down not long after, we brought the training over to a 100% online platform and have been working with yoga teachers all around the world since then, both online and in person. And now I am delighted to see Mental Health Aware Yoga graduates bringing the knowledge from the training into their regular yoga classes and into more specialized settings, like rehab centres, schools, mental health facilities and with survivors of domestic violence. And yoga teachers who are also psychologists and other mental health professionals are using this work to bring yoga into therapy.

My vision is to set a gold standard in mental health education for yoga teachers worldwide, to make yoga classes safe, nourishing and transformative for *all* yoga students, and we are just getting started on this audacious goal!

And now you have this book in your hands, I am delighted that you are part of this vision too.

WHY YOGA TEACHERS NEED TO KNOW ABOUT MENTAL HEALTH

We are all affected by mental health.

Chances are you know someone whose life has been affected by depression, anxiety or trauma, whether that is a friend, family member or a yoga student.

Perhaps that person is you.

In the Mental Health Aware Yoga training, I often begin the course by asking the attendees to not only share their name and intention for the training, but also their experience with mental health and mental illness. By the end of this ice-breaking exercise, it is always really clear how prevalent mental health challenges are. I have never heard anyone in the group say that they have never met anyone, in their personal or work life, who has not experienced mental health challenges. But it is often a surprise to the group. We so rarely share about mental illness, that it is easy to think that we are the only ones wrestling with it.

But we are not. And the statistics confirm it.

Nearly half the population report experiencing a diagnosable mental illness at some point in their life. This varies across countries and survey methods, but is true in Australia (45%),[2] the United Kingdom (43.4%)[3] and the USA (46.4%).[4] When we look at a 12-month period, the research tells us that one in five people have experienced a diagnosable mental illness in the past 12 months.[5]

The research usually only takes into consideration those who meet diagnostic criteria for a mental illness and does not include those who are feeling low, or who are struggling but do not meet the clinical cut-off point for a diagnosis or who do not ask for help. Therefore, it is likely that the rate of people experiencing mental health challenges is much higher.

Mental health issues are now considered to be one of the main causes of the overall disease burden worldwide, and major depression is considered to be the second leading cause of disability worldwide.[6] I think it is fairly safe to say that mental illness is a common experience.

In a landmark study in Australia back in 2005, Stephen Penman surveyed 3832 yoga students and teachers for his PhD thesis (myself included!) and found that 58.4% of yoga students began yoga to reduce stress or anxiety and 79.4% of yoga students continued to practise yoga to reduce stress or anxiety.[7] He suggested that mental health may be the primary health reason people practise yoga.

And with the rise of yoga and what seems to be a rise in the willingness talk about and seek support for mental health challenges, it is likely that this is even higher now. I would love to see another study done on this topic.

All this research confirms what many of us know to be true: that many people are struggling with the challenges of being human and are coming to yoga to seek refuge, support and a pathway home to their true selves.

I am glad you are here.

WHAT ROLE DO YOGA TEACHERS HAVE IN MENTAL HEALTH?

With so many people practising yoga for mental health reasons, yoga teachers have ended up at the frontline of contemporary mental health care, and now, more than ever, need to know how to support their students experiencing mental health challenges.

But yoga teachers are not therapists.

And yoga is not the cure for all of our problems.

To be clear, yoga is best practised alongside other lifestyle, psychological or pharmaceutical methods to support health, happiness and healing. Yoga provides a wonderful toolkit and road map for navigating life, but it is not enough on its own.

For those experiencing mild or sub-clinical levels of mental illness or distress, yoga may be used in conjunction with other lifestyle factors, such as nutrition, sleep, social connection, rest and living a life of purpose and meaning.

For those with moderate to severe levels of mental illness or distress, yoga may be a great adjunct to psychological and/or pharmaceutical therapies (as well as, of course, other lifestyle factors). It is important, I believe, that yoga is used in conjunction with these modalities, not to replace them.

So how can yoga teachers support their students' mental health?

Great question!

Yoga offers a veritable treasure trove of practices that are helpful for regulating the nervous system to create calm, clarity and equilibrium. Have you ever been to a yoga class feeling pretty overwhelmed by your life or the state of the world, and left feeling lighter than when you started? Or used a prāṇāyāma practice to help regulate your breath when you were feeling anxious?

This is the power of yoga practices.

But that is not all. The yoga class is a place where students can come and feel safe, seen and heard, without the stigma (perceived or otherwise) of being a client in therapy. Therapy is often an important part of recovery, but connecting with oneself and one's community outside of talk therapy is important too. And, for many, a yoga class can be a wonderful and often very healing way to do this. It is important not to underestimate this effect!

However, yoga teachers are not therapists. We are trained to teach yoga, not to provide counselling or medical advice, and it is important that we are clear about this and are mindful of our scope of practice. However, yoga teachers are what Gerard Egan calls *informal helpers*.[8] Informal helpers are professionals, like teachers, doctors, managers and lawyers, who are trained in their specific field, yet are still called on to support people through times of crisis or distress.

Yoga practices and the safe container in which yoga teachers hold their classes can be nourishing and supportive for students, and it is not uncommon for students to practise yoga for these very reasons. It is also not uncommon for students to start to open up about their challenges in the safe space that is created in the class and with their teacher.

We will touch more on scope of practice and referring to other health professionals later in the book, but, for now, it is safe to say that, as a yoga teacher, it is likely that you will be called on to be of support, and it is important to have the skills to do this.

If you are a yoga teacher and a mental health professional, which I am delighted to see more and more, then you are very well placed to integrate yoga into your counselling or clinical work, and you will find many ways to do this in this book.

COMPASSIONATE REFLECTION

1. What are your experiences with mental health and mental illness?
2. What have your personal highs and lows been?
3. In the past, what has helped your mental health when you were struggling?
4. What do you know helps to maintain positive mental health for you?
5. How have yoga teachings and practices helped your mental health?

Pillar One

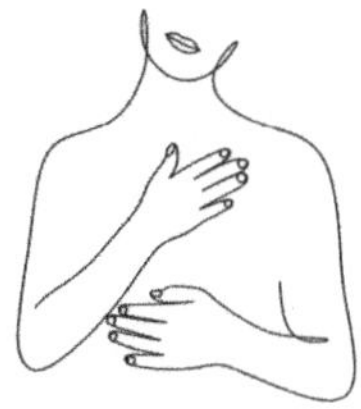

INTRODUCTION TO WESTERN PSYCHOLOGY

OVERVIEW

Over the last couple of decades, I have noticed a shift from many people not wanting to be put in a box with a diagnosis to, more recently, actively seeking out a diagnosis from a clinical psychologist or psychiatrist to make sense of their internal experience.

I wonder if this change is partly due to a reduction in stigma around mental illness as more and more people are speaking openly about their mental health challenges, and partly due to the more compassionate and nuanced conversations that are happening in the mental health space. No longer does a diagnosis of anxiety, depression or trauma mean that you are *going crazy* or that there is something wrong with you. Rather these diagnoses often reflect a very appropriate response to life's sometimes overwhelming challenges.

Whether you believe that a diagnosis is a helpful tool or not, I believe that it is important that you understand the language of diagnosis, so when a yoga student tells you about their recent diagnosis of social anxiety disorder or complex posttraumatic stress disorder, you understand what they are talking about and have an idea of how you can design a yoga class to support their needs.

In this chapter, we will be taking a look at mental illness through the lens of Western psychology, drawing on the diagnostic criteria outlined in the *Diagnostic and Statistical Manual of Mental Disorders (DSM-V)*[1] a publication by the American Psychiatric Association used by psychologists and psychiatrists to diagnose mental illness. We go into a lot more details about diagnosis in the Mental Health Aware Yoga training, but this chapter will give you a great overview.

To be clear, as a yoga teacher, it is not your job to diagnose or treat mental illness; however, as depression, anxiety, stress and trauma are so prevalent in our communities, I believe that it is important to understand the language of mental illness and understand the signs and symptoms, so we know what to look for in our students and understand how we can help.

DEPRESSION

Depression is characterized by a significantly low mood and loss of interest or pleasure in activities that were previously considered enjoyable.

Having a depressed mood some of the time is considered within the *normal* range of human experience; however, when this low mood state affects the quality of our life and continues for more than a couple of weeks, it may meet diagnostic criteria for major depression or another depressive disorder.

With 15% of people diagnosed with a depressive disorder in their lifetime,[2] depression is a remarkably common experience.

Symptoms of depression

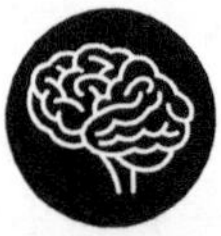	PSYCHOLOGICAL Sadness, feeling worthless, feeling helpless, feeling hopeless, guilt, thoughts of death or *negative* thoughts (e.g. 'I am not good enough' or 'I am unlovable').
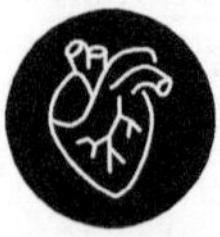	PHYSICAL Difficulty sleeping, feeling tired, weight loss or weight gain, or change in appetite.
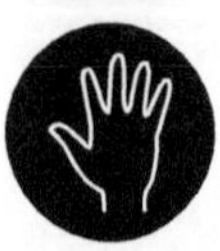	BEHAVIOURAL Lacking motivation, not wanting to go out, not wanting to engage in enjoyable activities anymore, frequent crying or difficulty concentrating.

Major depression

Major depression is often what we think about when we hear about a diagnosis of depression.

It can feel like going into a deep, dark cave for extended periods of time. Some people will live in this cave for a few weeks, others for a few years. It can be a difficult place to live.

To be diagnosed with major depression there must be a significant number of depressive symptoms, like the ones mentioned above, that significantly affect the quality of life and last for two weeks or more.

Persistent depressive disorder

Persistent depressive disorder, previously known as dysthymia, is a low-grade, long-term depression. It is chronic rather than acute.

Life with persistent depressive disorder can feel pretty grey and bland, with no hope in sight. However, as the symptoms are milder than major depressive disorder and as most people can continue to get on with life while experiencing it, it can be easily missed.

To be diagnosed with persistent depressive disorder, there must be a number of depressive symptoms, like the ones mentioned above, that have been present over at least a two-year period.

What depression looks like in a yoga class

Depression looks and feels different for everyone, but indicators that a yoga student *might* be depressed include:

- seeming sad most of the time
- crying
- a predominance of tamasic energy (we will explore this in the Yoga Psychology chapter)
- a hunched over posture, with stooped shoulders and a collapsed chest
- moving and speaking slowly
- sighing heavily or looking like they are barely breathing

- frequently running late to class
- feeling that they are not good enough and communicating this through their body language or the way they speak to themselves or others
- giving up easily in challenging postures
- feeling disheartened and hopeless if they do not get the postures *right*
- feeling exhausted
- feeling overwhelmed
- lacking motivation
- not interacting with other students
- having difficulty following your instructions or becoming easily confused
- poor body image
- hiding at the back of the class
- suddenly stopping coming to class
- being drawn to Śavāsana (Corpse Pose) or other restorative postures.

This list is merely intended to give you an idea of how a student with depression might show up in your yoga class. Presenting with just one or two of these indicators does not mean that your student is depressed. By the same token, if they do not exhibit any of these indicators, it does not mean that they are not depressed.

ANXIETY

Anxiety is characterized by excessive worry, rumination, physical sensations of fight-or-flight and avoidance of situations that cause anxiety.

Like all emotions, anxiety is part of the experience of being human and can help us to navigate, process and understand the world and ourselves. Moderate levels of anxiety can actually improve performance, and sometimes severe levels of anxiety can be experienced as normal when they are consistent with the demands of the situation.[3]

But anxiety disorders are more than just feeling a little anxious. The anxiety in anxiety disorders is irrational, results in avoidance of situations and can impact greatly on our lives.

With 26.3% of people diagnosed with an anxiety disorder in their lifetime, including 5.9% with generalized anxiety disorder, 10.6% with social anxiety disorder and 5.2% with panic disorder,[4] anxiety is a very common experience.

Symptoms of anxiety

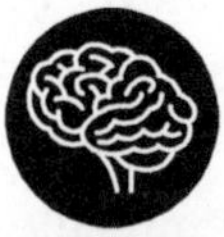	PSYCHOLOGICAL Excessive fear, worry, *negative* thoughts, catastrophizing, rumination or obsessive thinking.
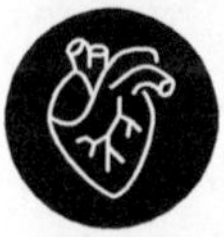	PHYSICAL Panic attacks, hot and cold flushes, racing heart, tightening of the chest, shallow rapid breathing, difficulty sleeping, restlessness or feeling tense, wound up and edgy.
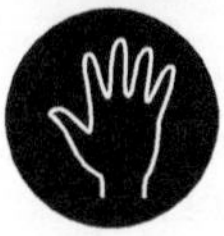	BEHAVIOURAL Avoidance of situations that arouse anxiety which can impact on study, work or social life.

Generalized anxiety disorder

Individuals with generalized anxiety disorder (GAD) are worried much of the time about a broad variety of things; they worry that disaster will occur despite their constant worrying. Individuals with GAD are often described by their loved ones as *worrying about everything* and it can seem like there is no end to the things to worry about.

To be diagnosed with generalized anxiety disorder, there must be excessive and largely uncontrollable anxiety and worry about a broad number of events or activities, occurring more days than not for at least six months.

Social anxiety disorder

Individuals with social anxiety disorder, or social phobia, fear negative evaluation in social situations. As a result, they often avoid social situations that trigger anxiety, which can paradoxically reinforce their anxiety and have a significant impact on their work and social life.

To be diagnosed with social anxiety disorder, there must be significant fear or anxiety about social situations and subsequent avoidance (or endurance with great difficulty) for at least six months.

Panic disorder

Individuals with panic disorder experience recurrent and unexpected panic attacks, and they worry about the implications of a panic attack and that they might happen again.

A panic attack is an abrupt surge of intense fear or discomfort that reaches a peak within minutes, and includes symptoms that can feel very scary, like heart palpitations, sweating, shaking, shortness of breath, chest pain, nausea, dizziness, numbness, feelings of unreality (derealization) or feeling detached from oneself (depersonalization), fear of *going crazy* or of dying. Many people who experience a panic attack for the first time call an ambulance or later visit their medical doctor, as the sensations of a panic attack can feel like a medical emergency.

With panic disorder, after a panic attack, there is a persistent worry about having another panic attack or about the consequences of another panic attack (like losing control, having a heart attack or *going crazy*), and a significant change in behaviour related to the attacks, like avoiding places or people in order to avoid having another panic attack.[5]

To be diagnosed with panic disorder, at least one of the panic attacks must have been followed by at least one month of persistent worry about additional panic attacks or their consequences or significant maladaptive changes in behaviour related to the attacks, like avoidance of possible triggers.

What anxiety looks like in a yoga class

Anxiety looks and feels different for everyone; however, some indicators that a yoga student *might* be experiencing anxiety include:

- appearing anxious, wound up or worried
- a predominance of rajasic energy (we will explore this in the Yoga Psychology chapter)
- moving and speaking quickly
- holding tension in their face and body
- breathing fast and shallow, or holding their breath
- arriving early for class
- looking around the room to see what others are doing
- being perfectionistic, striving to get postures *right*
- feeling frustrated or worried if they do not get postures *right*
- asking lots of questions
- looking restless in class, particularly in Śavāsana (Corpse Pose) and restorative postures
- being drawn to more dynamic styles, postures and movements.

As with depression, presenting with just one or two of these indicators does not mean that your student is anxious. Equally, if they do not exhibit any of these indicators, it does not mean that they are not anxious. This list is merely intended to give you an idea of how a student might show up in your yoga class if they are anxious.

TRAUMA

Trauma occurs as a result of powerlessness in the face of an overwhelming force when the ordinary systems that give us a sense of control, meaning and connection are overridden.[6]

By definition, trauma is unbearable and intolerable. As survivors of trauma often become understandably upset when they think about what they experienced, they often try to avoid situations that elicit the memory, pushing it out of their minds and acting as if nothing happened, which requires tremendous energy and resources.[7]

The experience of trauma is unfortunately a common one. In the USA, more than half of the population (and slightly more men than women) reported exposure to at least one traumatic incident in their lifetime, including rape, molestation, physical attack, combat, shock, threat with a weapon, accidents, natural disasters, abuse, neglect or witnessing something traumatic.[8]

In a Norwegian study, 91% of patients in a psychiatric hospital reported being exposed to at least one traumatic incident in their lives, and 69% of patients reported being repeatedly exposed to trauma over longer periods of time.[9]

However, not everyone who experiences a traumatic incident develops posttraumatic stress disorder (PTSD).[10] The proportion of people diagnosed with PTSD in their lifetime is 12.2%.[11] But just because someone is not diagnosed with PTSD, does not mean that they do not feel the effects of a traumatic experience.

Several years ago, I was in the Bourke Street Mall in Melbourne, Australia, with my young children when a man drove his car down the pedestrian mall killing and injuring many people. It seemed like the entire downtown Melbourne stopped in its tracks, with injured people lying on the street, crowds of people huddled together looking on in confusion from the eaves of the shops, helicopters overhead and police sirens filling the air. It was very scary. I had been in London when the bombs went off in the city in 2005, and the experience of confusion, helicopters and police sirens took me right back there. Until I learned later on the news what had happened, I thought we were in the middle of a terrorist attack.

My children and I were unharmed, but I felt the reverberation of the incident in my body for days and weeks afterwards. Thankfully, with years of yoga and psychology under my belt, I had the tools to meet the trauma, and while I am still not keen on returning to Bourke Street all these years later, I did not develop PTSD and barely think about what happened there anymore.

And yet, when I went to a yoga class about a year after the incident and the teacher instructed us to hold our arms above our head for a very long time, my arms began to ache and my body remembered the ache of holding my children in my arms and running away during the Bourke Street incident. I was no longer actively thinking about what had happened, but my body remembered it, and the memory was triggered in a yoga posture.

So does this mean that we should never ask our students to hold their arms above their head for an extended period of time in case they had an experience similar to mine?

No.

But it does mean we that we need to be aware that anything could potentially trigger a traumatic memory or experience, and it is important that we offer our students choice and respect their autonomy over their bodies.

Given the prevalence of trauma in our communities, and the far-reaching effects it can have on people's lives, it is vital that we do our best to make our yoga classes a safe and nurturing space for our students who have experienced trauma.

Symptoms of trauma

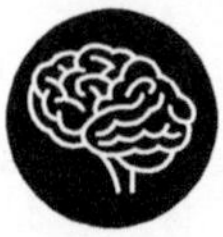	**PSYCHOLOGICAL** Recurrent and intrusive memories and/or flashbacks of a traumatic event, distressing dreams, feeling distressed if there is a reminder of the traumatic event, depression, fear, difficulty concentrating, dissociation, irritability, helplessness or feeling disconnected from self and others.
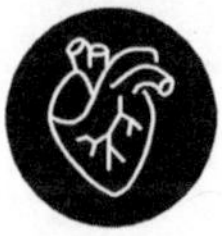	**PHYSICAL** Panic attacks, racing heart, fatigue, breathing quickly, mouth breathing, restlessness, feeling tense or wound up.
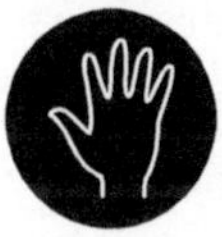	**BEHAVIOURAL** Avoidance of stimuli associated with the traumatic event, hypervigilance, decrease in social engagement, decrease engagement in previously enjoyable activities, exaggerated startle response, sleep dysregulation, reckless or self-destructive behaviour or angry outbursts.

Posttraumatic stress disorder

Posttraumatic stress disorder (PTSD) is what many of us think about when we think about the after effects of trauma, and this is the trauma diagnosis found in the *Diagnostic and Statistical Manual of Mental Disorders (DSM-V)*.[12]

To be diagnosed with PTSD, you must have experienced, witnessed or have someone close to you involved in serious injury, violence or death,[13] and, afterwards, experience a number of symptoms, including intrusive and distressing memories or dreams of the traumatic event, flashbacks in which it feels as if the traumatic event is happening again, distress when around experiences that are similar to the traumatic event, avoidance of people or things that arouse recollections of the traumatic event, hypervigilance, irritable and angry outbursts, difficulty concentrating or sleep disturbance.[14]

Complex posttraumatic stress disorder

Two influential trauma therapists, Dr Bessel van der Kolk[15] and Dr Judith Herman[16], have argued that the criteria for PTSD does not fully and accurately represent the full spectrum of the traumatic experience and ensuing suffering, particularly for those who have experienced prolonged and repeated trauma, such as childhood abuse or domestic violence.

In her book *Trauma and Recovery*, Judith proposes a new way of looking at trauma, which she calls complex posttraumatic stress disorder.

Complex posttraumatic stress disorder (C-PTSD) may occur after an extended period of 'totalitarian control', such as domestic abuse, childhood physical or sexual abuse, being held hostage, serving as a prisoner of war, surviving concentration camps, enduring certain religious cults or experiencing organized sexual exploitation.[17]

The symptoms of C-PTSD, which can occur following prolonged traumatic incidents, include changes in mood regulation, a sense of unease or dissatisfaction with life, chronic suicidal thoughts, self-injury, explosive or inhibited anger, compulsive or extremely inhibited sexuality, memory loss or a vivid memory of traumatic experiences, sense of helpless and hopelessness, feelings of shame, guilt and self-blame, social withdrawal, persistent distrust and repeated failures of self-protection.[18] This is sometimes diagnosed as borderline personality disorder.[19,20]

What trauma looks like in a yoga class

Trauma can look and feel different for everyone; however, indicators that a yoga student *might* be experiencing PTSD or C-PTSD include:

- symptoms of depression or anxiety
- a predominance of rajasic and/or tamasic energy
- being constantly on alert and looking around the class
- jumping in response to loud sounds (e.g. a door slamming)
- keeping eyes open in class, including during meditation and relaxation
- holding tension in the body and face
- looking restless
- difficulty trusting others
- seeming uncomfortable when a new teacher covers the class without warning
- seeming uncomfortable when a class is significantly different from previous classes
- daydreaming or dissociating (not being present or getting stuck in a posture)
- not wanting to be touched or receive hands-on assists
- not wanting to do partner work
- seeming uncomfortable when the lights are dimmed
- leaving during the class
- not engaging with others.

Again, presenting with just one or two of these indicators does not mean that your student has experienced trauma. By the same token, if they do not exhibit any of these indicators, it does not mean that they have not experienced trauma. This list is merely intended to give you an idea of how a student might show up in your yoga class if they have an experience of trauma that continues to affect them.

STRESS

Stress occurs when the challenges of life exceed our ability to cope with them.

A survey by the Australian Psychological Society found that 35% of people reported having significant distress in their lives, with 14% reporting mild distress, 8% reporting moderate distress and 13% reporting experiencing severe levels of distress.[21] In the study, the top five causes of stress included personal finances, family issues, personal health, trying to maintain a healthy lifestyle and issues with the health of others close to us. Sound familiar?

While stress is not listed in the *DSM-V* as a mental illness, it does significantly affect our mental health and is likely to be commonly experienced by many of your yoga students.

Symptoms of stress

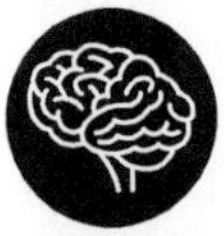	**PSYCHOLOGICAL** Feeling overwhelmed, worry, fear, anger, tearfulness, irritability, anxiety, helplessness or memory problems.
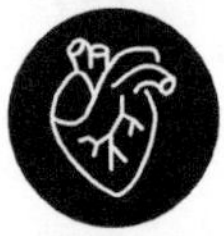	**PHYSICAL** Heart palpitations, fatigue, stomach upset, diarrhoea, headaches, muscular aches and pains, weakened immune system or high blood pressure.
	**Behavioural** Difficulty concentrating, fatigue, lacking motivation, sleep disturbance, insomnia, social withdrawal, unhealthy eating habits or short temper.

A definition of stress

A *stressor* is anything that affects our wellbeing or survival, and *stress* is a natural human response to a stressor designed to bring us back to homeostasis (the way in which the body maintains its internal equilibrium for wellbeing and survival).

A stressor can be an external threat, like a global pandemic or losing your job, or it can be internal, like feeling time-pressured or worried about the way that you are perceived by your friends.

We can also think about stress as either acute or chronic.

Mild acute stress, like starting a new job or giving a presentation, can lead to developing an adaptive response to meeting life's challenges; but severe stress, like being exposed to a violent and life-threatening crime, can lead to PTSD or other mental health challenges.

Chronic stress, on the other hand, is stress that continues over an extended period of time, such as chronic health issues, relationship difficulties, financial problems, bullying, social isolation or living in an unsafe environment. This can also result in mental illness.

The stress response and the nervous system

The stress response activates the autonomic nervous system, the part of the nervous system that is in charge of bodily functions but is not under our conscious control. There are three main branches of the autonomic nervous system: the sympathetic, the parasympathetic and the enteric.

The sympathetic branch is activated during the stress response and is like an accelerator in a car, triggering the *fight-or-flight* response and providing the body with a burst of energy to respond to perceived dangers. The parasympathetic branch, on the other hand, promotes the *rest-and-digest* response and is more like the brake in the car, dampening the stress response once the threat has passed.[22]

The enteric branch of the nervous system is not widely discussed, but actually has a similar number of neurons as the spinal cord and is sometimes called the *little brain*.[23] The enteric nervous system is embedded in the lining of the gut, orchestrates various digestive functions and is adversely affected by stress.[24]

When the sympathetic branch of the autonomic nervous system kicks in, it prepares us to meet the stressor; dilating our pupils, speeding up our heart, slowing down our digestion and raising our blood pressure.

Activation of the sympathetic nervous system has an important role and is designed to save our lives in times of crisis, but, if it is triggered too often, it can result in stress-related diseases, including mental health problems, cardiovascular disease, obesity, gastrointestinal problems and more.

Is stress all bad?

Stress has a bad reputation, but a little bit of stress can actually be a good thing. It can help to keep us alive when we are in danger and it can actually improve our performance.

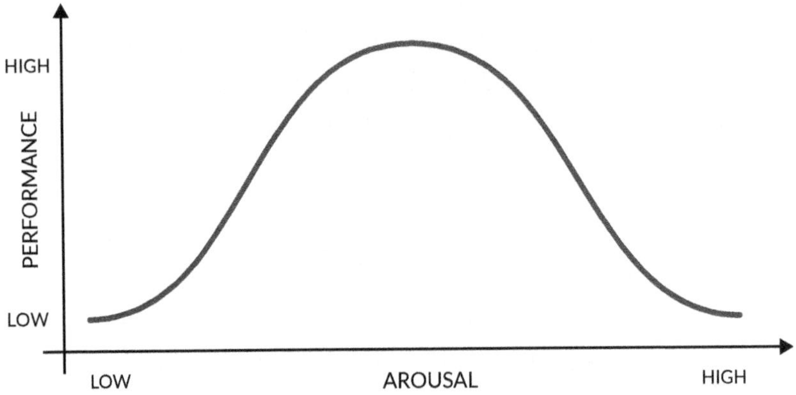

YERKES-DODSON LAW

Based on Yerkes and Dodson's experiments with mice in 1908,[25] the Yerkes-Dodson Law states that arousal (stress) improves performance up to a certain point, then performance reduces as arousal increases, particularly with more difficult tasks.[26] Optimal performance is achieved with a moderate amount of arousal, but not so much that it tips us into overwhelm.

Responses to stress

There are three typical responses to stress based on the severity of the stress and our capacity to respond:[27]

	The stressor and the individual's ability to respond are *well-matched* and the response results in a *return to balance or homeostasis*. This is likely to be a less severe or threatening stressor.

	The stressor may be excessive or continual and be *greater than the individual's capacity* to respond. This is likely to be a more severe or ongoing stressor, and results in *vulnerability* as a result of stress.
	While the stressor may be excessive or ongoing, there is a *good match* between the stressor and the individual's capacity to respond, leading to *posttraumatic growth* or anti-fragility. This is not always discussed in relation to stress and trauma, but can be an important and powerful catalyst for growth and developing inner strength and wisdom.

While I believe that is important to recognize and celebrate posttraumatic growth and our potential for growth through adversity, it is also important to acknowledge that extreme stress does not always result in growth.

What does not kill does not always make us stronger. Sometimes it makes us more vulnerable. I say this not to bring the party down, but to remind ourselves that being human can be a complex thing, and there is no shame if you have been through a traumatic event and you are still feeling the aftershocks of your experience, months, years or decades later.

What stress looks like in a yoga class

Stress looks and feels different for everyone; however, indicators that a yoga student *might* be stressed include:

- symptoms of depression, anxiety or trauma
- a predominance of rajasic and/or tamasic energy
- crying
- holding tension in their face and body
- nervous behaviours, like biting nails, pacing and fidgeting
- frequently running late
- frequently unwell
- difficulty concentrating
- feeling exhausted

- feeling overwhelmed
- feeling irritable
- not interacting with other students
- giving up easily in challenging postures
- feeling disheartened and hopeless if they do not get the postures *right*
- not following your instructions or easily confused
- stops coming to class
- has difficulty relaxing.

Note that presenting with just one or two of these indicators does not mean that your student is stressed. And on the same note, if they do not exhibit any of these indicators, it does not mean that they are not feeling stressed. This list is merely intended to give you an idea of how a student might show up in a yoga class if they are feeling stressed.

It is interesting to note how much overlap there is between the indicators and symptoms for depression, anxiety, stress and trauma. Which brings us to our next topic on co-morbidity!

CO-MORBIDITY

While we commonly speak about discrete categories of mental illness, the reality is that they frequently occur together.

One study in the Netherlands found that in individuals with a current depressive disorder, 67% also had a current anxiety disorder and 81% had experienced an anxiety disorder in their lifetime.[28] In those with a current anxiety disorder, they found that 63% had a current depressive disorder and 81% had experienced a depressive disorder at some point in their lifetime.[29]

In individuals with a diagnosis of PTSD, over 80% are also diagnosed with another mental disorder or medical illness, including co-morbidity with anxiety, depression, substance abuse, personality disorders and medical illness.[30]

Why this is important to know

If a student has a diagnosis of one particular mental illness, or they present with symptoms of one, it is fairly likely that they will also have symptoms or even meet the diagnostic criteria of another.

In my experience, individuals with depression often also have symptoms of anxiety, people with ongoing anxiety often get depressed, and those with a history of trauma often show symptoms of either (or both) depression and anxiety. In addition, stress can lead to mental illness and mental illness can be pretty stressful to live with.

It is safe to say that there is a significant overlap and co-occurrence of mental illness using this Western model of diagnosis and there is no one-size-fits-all approach that works for everyone based on their diagnosis.

What does this mean for yoga teachers?

So far, we have looked at four distinct diagnostic categories: depression, anxiety, trauma and stress, but we can see from the lists of symptoms I have included in this chapter and the way they may present in the context of a yoga class that there is a lot of overlap.

The good news is we can draw on the tradition of yoga and take a different approach to understanding our student's mental health, through the lens of the guṇas.

But more on this in the next chapter!

COMPASSIONATE REFLECTION

1. Did you identify personally with any of the symptoms or diagnostic criteria in this chapter?
2. Is there anything that you need to do to support yourself after reading this chapter?
3. After reading about the symptoms of depression, anxiety, stress and trauma and how they present in a yoga class, do any of your students come to mind?

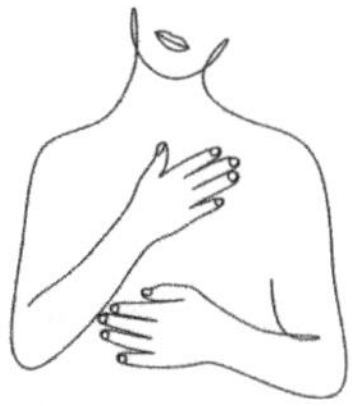

Pillar Two

FOUNDATIONS OF YOGA PSYCHOLOGY

WHAT IS YOGA?

Commentaries on the meaning of the word *yoga* vary from union, to attaining what was previously unattainable, to directing all our focus on the activity in which we are engaged, to being one with the divine.[1]

The meaning of *yoga* is presented concisely in Patañjali's Yoga Sūtras, a text that is considered by many to be the heart of yoga.[2]

Chapter 1, verse 2 of the Yoga Sūtras states:

yogaś citta vṛtti nirodhaḥ (I.2)

Different commentators have interpreted this sutra in many subtly different ways:

'*Yoga is the ability to direct the mind exclusively toward an object and sustain that direction without any distractions.*' T.K.V. Desikachar[3]

'*Yoga is the cessation of movements in the consciousness.*' B.K.S. Iyengar[4]

'*Yoga is the stilling of the changing states of mind.*' Edwin F. Bryant[5]

'*Yoga is the restriction of the whirls of consciousness.*' Georg Feuerstein[6]

'*Yoga is the cessation of the modification of consciousness.*' Anand Mehrotra[7]

'*Yoga is the calming of the fluctuations of the mind in order to find unity within.*' Susanna Barkataki[8]

> '*Yoga is when we knowingly live as the realization of unconditioned Stillness, whether thought is in movement or stillness.*' Richard Miller[9]

However you translate and interpret this most influential sūtra, it is clear that yoga is related to the mind and self-understanding, and not to having a slim and flexible body that looks sexy in an expensive, tight-fitting outfit.

But you already knew that, didn't you?

In this chapter on yoga psychology, we will explore this further by looking at Patañjali's eight limbs of yoga, as well as the guṇas and the koshas.

EIGHT LIMBS OF PATAÑJALI'S YOGA SŪTRAS

Patañjali's Yoga Sūtras

I am sure you remember Patañjali's Yoga Sūtras from your very first yoga teacher training course, and have probably referred back to them many times since.

Patañjali's Yoga Sūtras are a timeless and practical psycho-social-somatic-spiritual guide to understanding ourselves and the world, overcoming suffering and realizing enlightenment.

While little is known about Patañjali himself, it is widely accepted that he was an authority on yoga and compiled and systemized the Vedic knowledge of the time into 196 sūtras that could be handed down orally from teacher to student, in a way that was concise and therefore possible to remember.[10]

These sūtras comprise a series of experiments or practices that were designed to realize the teachings of Sāṅkhya, teachings which can be traced back to 2500 BCE in lands that are now known as India and Iran,[11] although some claim the teachings can be traced back thousands of years earlier.[12]

The Sāṅkhya dualistic philosophy states that the seer (*Puruṣa*) and the seen (*Prakṛiti*) are separate constructs, and is the framework in which Advaita, Kashmir Shaivism and Buddhism were built upon.[13]

It is estimated that Patañjali compiled the sūtras around the second century CE (year 101–200) and that Vyāsa wrote the original commentary on the sūtras, *Yoga-Bhâshya*, around the fifth century CE (year 401–500).[14]

Within the Yoga Sūtras, Patañjali shared eight limbs, otherwise known as Ashtanga Yoga:

> Yama-niyamāsana-prāṇāyāma-pratyāhāra-dhāraṇā-dhyāna-dhyāna-samādhayo 'ṣṭāv aṅgāni (II.29)[15]

The eight limbs form the foundation of the practice and realization of yoga. They include:

1. Yamas (guidance for engaging with the world)
2. Niyamas (guidance for engaging with ourselves)
3. Asana (postures)
4. Prāṇāyāma (breath control and regulation)
5. Pratyāhāra (awareness or withdrawal of the senses)
6. Dhāraṇā (one-pointed concentration)
7. Dhyāna (meditation or contemplation)
8. Samādhi (oneness with everything).

Let's now explore these eight limbs through the lens of Mental Health Aware Yoga.

YAMAS

> Ahiṁsā-satyāsteya-brahmacaryāparigrahā yamāḥ (II.30)[16]

The five yamas: ahiṁsā, satya, asteya, brahmacarya and aparigraha, relate to our relationship with the world. They guide us to live in the world in a way that cultivates sattva (clarity, wisdom and happiness) in ourselves and others, in order to obtain self-realization.

Ahiṁsā

Ahiṁsā translates to mean *non-violence,* and relates to thinking and acting in ways that are kind and thoughtful to all living creatures.

Ahiṁsā requires thoughtful consideration, and is not a precept we can mindlessly follow.

Some commentaries indicate that ahiṁsā includes not eating meat, or even not eating root vegetables, as farming may result in the harm of creatures in the soil,[17] but others allow for some flexibility and state that ahiṁsā does not necessarily mean that we need to be vegetarian or that we cannot defend ourselves if we need to.[18]

I am a long-time vegetarian. When I was experiencing some health issues a few years ago, it was suggested to me by several practitioners that eating meat might be helpful, and was appropriate from a yogic and ayurvedic perspective as it was required for health reasons. My Buddhist acupuncturist pointed out, when she was trying to convince me to eat meat, that even the Dalai Lama ate meat when his doctors told him he needed to for his health. In the end, after much soul searching, I decided to try eating meat again to see if it helped improve my health. My health did not improve from eating meat, so the experiment did not last long, but I did come to a new understanding of ahiṁsā and I knew that I had tried everything to improve my health, even if it was outside my comfort zone.

Ahiṁsā is arguably *the* most important consideration when supporting the mental health of our students. There are very many āsana and prāṇāyāma practices to regulate the nervous system and support positive mental health, but it is unlikely that any of these will help if ahiṁsā is not present.

As Mental Health Aware Yoga teachers, we can cultivate ahiṁsā in our classes by being kind to our students, creating a safe and nourishing container to teach in, teaching yoga practices and sequences that are nourishing and invitational rather than forceful or dogmatic and doing our best not to cause harm. We will go into much more detail about all of these things in the Safe Container and Yogic Practices chapters of the book.

And as our students are just as likely to notice *how* we show up in class as well as *what* we actually *say*, it is extra important that we practise ahiṁsā for ourselves, being kind, compassionate and thoughtful towards ourselves too.

Satya

Satya translates to mean *truthfulness* or *non-lying.*

This includes honesty with ourselves and with others, and living in a way that is genuine, authentic and in integrity.

As Mental Health Aware Yoga teachers, it is important that we examine our own motivations and biases, and seek to live and teach in a way that is honest, authentic and in alignment with our values.

When teaching, instead of telling your students what they should or should not do, try encouraging them to find the answers within, to find their own truth and their own way of practising that feels right for them.

There is a lot of misinformation about yoga and mental health, especially online and on social media. Before you make any claims about yoga and mental health and add to the noise, be sure to check if your information is coming from a reputable source and that it rings true for you.

Like ahiṁsā, satya is a concept that requires consideration, compassion and thoughtfulness, not blind obedience, and it is important to keep ahiṁsā in mind and consider refraining (or reframing) a *truth* that may be harmful to another.

Asteya

Asteya is widely translated to mean *not stealing* or *honesty.*

This includes not stealing others' belongings, but it is also means not taking others' ideas and presenting them as our own, not imitating others' style of living[19] and not betraying someone's confidence when they have confided in us.[20]

Asteya goes beyond simply not stealing. When we commit to honesty and not stealing from others, we can celebrate and appreciate what we have, rather than feeling jealous and unworthy in comparison with others, and, in doing so, let go of our attachments to a small sense of self and connect to something greater.[21] The realization of asteya is that nothing is owned by us anyway.[22]

Personally, I have found that practising asteya brings peace of mind. If I have done something where I fear getting caught out, then it sits uncomfortably with me and I feel a heavy weight on my shoulders. I find life is much more enjoyable and stress-free when my conscience is clear. And when I can let go of the aching for what others have that I do not and be content and grateful with my life as it is, I feel such a sense of freedom and gratitude.

As Mental Health Aware Yoga teachers, we can practise asteya by finding our own unique way of teaching and sharing the wisdom of yoga, by crediting the wisdom and knowledge of others when we share from other sources, by standing up against abuse and exploitation of others and by practicing gratitude and appreciation for what is already in our lives.

I have been mindful of asteya in this book, in which I have carefully referenced other people's ideas and translations throughout, even though it might feel a little cumbersome for the reader at times.

Brahmacarya

Brahmacarya is often translated to mean *celibacy* or *chastity*, but is more than simply abstaining from sexual activity.

T.K.V. Desikachar states 'brahmacarya suggests that we should form relationships that foster our understanding of the highest truths. If sensual pleasures are part of those relationships, we must take care that we keep our direction and do not get lost.'[23]

Whether we choose to abstain from sexual relationships or not, as Mental Health Aware Yoga teachers, it is important that we are mindful of our sexual energy and do not bring it into the student–teacher relationship. This includes avoiding flirting, sexual innuendo, sexualized behaviour or sexual relationships with students and avoiding using sexual imagery as a marketing strategy to attract students to our classes. Not only is this not in alignment with brahmacarya, but it could also feel very unsafe for some students, including those who have experienced sexual abuse. We will explore this more in the Safe Container chapter.

Susanna Barkataki, the author of *Embrace Yoga's Roots*, shares a broader understanding of brahmacarya for householders, those of us who are engaged in the world with study, families and careers. She describes brahmacarya as energy management, such that we use our life force energy for higher spiritual purposes, rather than simply satisfying our individual desires.[24]

As Mental Health Aware Yoga teachers, we can consciously and intentionally use our energy to cultivate conditions conducive to healing, happiness and awakening for ourselves, our students, our families and our communities.

Aparigraha

Aparigraha translates to *non-grasping* or *non-attachment*, and means letting go of possessiveness and the constant cycle of wanting more.

This does not necessarily mean that we do not have things that bring us joy, comfort or pleasure, but that we take only what is necessary and do not hold these things too tightly or define ourselves by them. After all, we are merely temporary caretakers of the possessions we accumulate in our lives.

As Mental Health Aware Yoga teachers, one way that we can cultivate aparigraha is to let go of our attachments to how things *should* be in our classes.

This relates to our teaching, as we allow ourselves to be the teacher that we already are, rather than comparing ourselves to other more experienced or more popular teachers. It also relates to the way we share yoga practices with our students, supporting them to take their focus inwards and practising yoga in a way that is right for them, rather than how they think they *should* be practising or comparing themselves to others in the class.

Many people, students and teachers alike, compare themselves endlessly to others and find themselves lacking. By modelling and gently encouraging our students to tune into their own internal compass, we can help them to reduce the focus on what they do not have and what they cannot do, and instead cultivate self-acceptance and appreciation.

Another way to practise aparigraha is to avoid *yoga consumerism* by being mindful of our choices of promoting brands or products in our studios or online and being intentional in the way we dress and consume products and brands ourselves. This is a way to cultivate self-acceptance and embody the understanding that happiness lies not in accumulating more stuff, but in simply being.

COMPASSIONATE REFLECTION

1. Which of these yamas are you already integrating into your life and teaching?
2. Were there any new ideas in this section on the yamas that you would like to bring into your life or work?
3. Try out one of these ideas in your teaching, then spend some time reflecting on how it went, including what went well, what did not go so well and what you would do differently next time.

NIYAMAS

Śauca-santoṣa-tapaḥ-svādhyāyeśvara-praṇidhānāni niyamāḥ (II.32)[25]

The five niyamas, śauca, saṃtoṣa, tapas, svādhyāya and īśvara-praṇidhānā, relate to self-regulation and guide us to cultivate sattva within ourselves and find enlightenment.

Śauca

Śauca is often translated to mean *cleanliness* or *purity*. It refers to keeping our environment clean, having good hygiene, a healthy body and clarity of mind.[26]

As Mental Health Aware Yoga teachers, one way that we can cultivate śauca externally is by keeping the space we teach in uncluttered and clean. This can be particularly helpful for those with sensory sensitivities and can have the internal effect of creating a space that is conducive to feeling calm and uncluttered. We will be exploring this in more detail in the Safe Container chapter.

We can also cultivate śauca on an internal level by practising and teaching yoga practices designed to increase sattva (clarity) and decrease rajas (agitation) and tamas (lethargy) in the body and mind. We will be exploring this in more detail in the Yogic Practices chapter.

Saṃtoṣa

Saṃtoṣa translates to mean *contentment.*

> 'True happiness comes from contentment with whatever one has, not with thinking that one will be happy when one gets all that one desires.'[27]

In a world that is constantly focused on doing more and having more, choosing contentment is a radical act and one that I believe has the power to change not only our internal experience but to disrupt the foundations of the capitalist society that we live in.

I have found that practising gratitude is a very practical way to cultivate contentment, and various studies have shown that having a daily practice can significantly affect our physical and emotional health.[28,29]

As Mental Health Aware Yoga teachers, we can model contentment in the way we engage with ourselves, and we can be intentional in our language while we are teaching yoga, supporting our students to be content with their practice just as it is and to find acceptance in each moment. We will be exploring language further in the Therapeutic Skills chapter.

To cultivate gratitude in a yoga class, you might invite your students at the beginning or end of class to take a moment to feel gratitude for themselves for taking this time out of their busy day to practise yoga, or to silently express gratitude for something or someone in their life. However, it is important that we are careful not to insist people feel grateful, as this could have the opposite effect and make someone feel worse. Instead, simply offer it as an invitation.

Tapas

Tapas is commonly translated to mean *austerity, self-discipline* or *perseverance.*

It involves cultivating an inner fire to help us to stay on track and achieve our spiritual goals.

In his commentary on the Sūtras, Georg Feuerstein cautioned that 'tapas must not be confused with harmful self-castigation and fakiristic self-torture.'[30] Similarly, T.K.V Desikachar said 'tapas must not cause suffering. That is very important.'[31] Tapas is not about creating unnecessary hardship for ourselves, but rather about passion, presence and self-mastery; 'whatever you are engaged in, you are engaged in it with the totality of your being'.[32]

Susanna Barkataki describes tapas as self-discipline that burns away impurities and kindles the fires of divinity, showing up in the choices we make and the struggle between 'I do not want to' and the 'I am going to do this'.[33] Have you ever woken up in the morning and felt warm and cosy in bed and not wanted to get up and do your morning yoga practice? I know I have! Tapas is when you get up and step onto your mat anyway, even when you do not really feel like it.

As Mental Health Aware Yoga teachers, one way that we can share tapas with our students is by gently encouraging them to show up for their practice on a regular basis, even just for one minute. One minute is often enough and, at times, is all that can be tolerated or made time for when times are tough.

Svādhyāya

Svādhyāya translates to mean *self-study* or *self-enquiry*, and involves looking internally to understand oneself and the world.

Svādhyāya is often translated to mean the study of ancient texts or the repetition of mantras. This is simply because both of these activities act as reference points in our self-study.[34] They are guidance on the path to self-enquiry and understanding, not the path itself.

You are engaging in svādhyāya by reading this book, journalling with the reflective prompts and by implementing the ideas you read here in your own life and teaching. But you are also engaging in svādhyāya by listening to your own needs about when to keep reading and when to take a break as you become tired, hungry or distracted and when to return to this book when the time is right for you.

As Mental Health Aware Yoga teachers, one way that we can foster svādhyāya in our students is by sharing wisdom from texts like Patañjali's Yoga Sūtras with them. Depending on the context that we are teaching in and the individual needs of the students, this might be sharing a passage from the Sūtras and talking about Patañjali, or it might simply be weaving themes like kindness (ahiṁsā) or contentment (saṃtoṣa) in the class without mentioning the Sūtras at all.

Another way we can bring svādhyāya into our teaching is by encouraging our students to compassionately and non-judgementally notice their internal experiences, listen to their own needs in each moment and practise in a way that is nourishing for them.

You might have noticed that there can be, at times, a tension between svādhyāya and tapas[35] when there is a discrepancy between our moment-by-moment needs and our greater spiritual or life goals. It requires wisdom and discernment to know when to listen to our needs in the moment and when to bring in the discipline to practice even when we do not feel like it.

Īśvarapraṇidhānā

Īśvarapraṇidhānā translates to mean *surrendering* oneself to God or a higher power.

If the idea of surrendering to a divine presence does not resonate with you, then another way to consider this niyama is *surrendering to the flow of life* or giving up our illusions of control.

As Mental Health Aware Yoga teachers, we can bring īśvarapraṇidhānā into our classes by inviting our students to be present in the moment, just as it is, and accept themselves just as they are, without trying to fix or change anything. It is a pretty simple idea, but it is not necessarily easy to do!

If it resonates for you and is appropriate in the context you are teaching in, consider threading in themes of surrendering to the flow of life, to a higher power or to God.

COMPASSIONATE REFLECTION

1. Which of these niyamas are you already integrating into your life and teaching?
2. Were there any new ideas in this section on the niyamas that you would like to bring into your life or work?

3. Pick one and try it out in your teaching, then spend some time reflecting on how it went, including what went well, what did not go so well and what you would do differently next time.

ĀSANA

Āsana translates to mean *postures* or *poses.* The goal of āsana is to allow the yogi to sit for meditation in a way that is steady and comfortable and does not disturb or distract the mind[36] in order to obtain self-realization.

While āsana is what is commonly considered to be the basis of yoga and where many people begin their yoga practice, āsana is actually given very little attention in Patañjali's Yoga Sūtras.

But this does not mean that it is not important.

Āsana can be a powerful vehicle to cultivate sattva and to explore themes of presence, mindfulness, self-compassion, interoception, embodiment, self-regulation and self-knowledge.

According to the Haṭha Yoga Pradīpikā, the role of āsana is to reduce rajas (agitation and anxiety) in order to cultivate sattva (clarity and wisdom).[37] Practising in a way that is steady and comfortable rather than forceful or arduous is an important part of this. Ideally, we want to practise āsana in a way that supports and nourishes us to carry out our dharma (the roles we play in our life) rather than detracting from it[38] and encourage our students to do the same.

This does not mean that we cannot practise or teach a dynamic or strong class, but that we practise this way only if it suits our body and constitution and aids us in cultivating sattva.

We will be exploring āsana for mental health in more depth in the Yogic Practices chapter.

PRĀṆĀYĀMA

The word *prāṇāyāma* is comprised of two parts: *prāṇā* and *āyāma. Prāṇā* is *that which is infinitely everywhere*, it is our vitality and continually flows from within us, filling us and keeping us alive. *Ayāma* means to *stretch* or *extend* and refers to the action of prāṇāyāma.[39]

Prāṇāyāma involves consciously focusing our attention on the breath.

We can practise prāṇāyāma to help us to understand ourselves, our state of mind and to shift our internal state from a predominance of rajas or tamas to a more sattvic state.

The breath can be a powerful tool for self-understanding, as the quality of our breath is closely linked to our state of mind. The breath is often faster, arrhythmic and shallow when we are anxious or agitated, and deeper, quieter and more rhythmic when we are relaxed and at ease. By noticing the breath, we can gain important insight into our mental health.

Once we have an understanding of our internal state, we can then utilize prāṇāyāma practices to shift it. Down-regulating or calming prāṇāyāma practices can be drawn upon when we are feeling more rajasic or anxious, and up-regulating or energizing prāṇāyāma practices can be utilized when tamas, lethargy or depression is present.

Like āsana, prāṇāyāma practices can also be a way to explore themes of presence, mindfulness, self-compassion, interoception and embodiment.

We will be exploring prāṇāyāma for mental health in more depth in the Yogic Practices chapter.

PRATYĀHĀRA

Pratyāhāra is the threshold between the internal and external practices of yoga.[40]

Ahāra means *nourishment*, so *pratyāhāra* translates as *to withdraw oneself from that which nourishes the senses*[41] and we can achieve this not by forcing ourselves not to look at something, but by focusing the mind on one specific thing so the senses are less likely to respond to other objects.

Pratyāhāra is a state that arises spontaneously, rather than a specific technique.[42] Like sleep, we cannot make it happen, but we can create conditions that are conducive for it to arise by giving the mind something to focus on.

In a yoga class, we might invite our students to focus their mind on a particular object, like the breath, a mantra or a specific drishti during āsana, and offer opportunities to close the eyes (or soften the gaze) and sense the body internally. While this can be beneficial for students experiencing mental health challenges, it can also be difficult, confusing and potentially triggering, so it is important to go gently and offer it only as an option, not as a requirement.

Not all students will be comfortable closing their eyes, and some people will feel unsafe if you ask this of them. So be sure to always give your students the option of eyes open or closed, or just leave out any instructions about what the eyes should be doing at all; students will likely come to their own conclusions about this. We will explore this more in the Safe Container chapter.

DHĀRAṆĀ, DHYĀNA AND SAMĀDHI

The five limbs discussed up until this point have been focused on preparing the mind, and now *dhāraṇā*, *dhyāna* and *samādhi* are the fruits of these five limbs.[43]

Dhāraṇā means *to hold* or *concentration* and is the ability to focus the mind on a single object, despite many potential distractions, and *dhyāna* is translated to mean *meditation* and is the state in which the mind has an uninterrupted flow or connection only in relation to the object it is focused on.[44,45]

Samādhi means *to bring together* or *to merge* and is a result of dhāraṇā and dhyāna. When the mind becomes so absorbed with an object that we become completely one with it, our personal identity completely disappears.[46]

While we cannot directly practise or teach dhāraṇā, dhyāna and samādhi, we can practise and teach āsana and prāṇāyāma to create optimal conditions for these three states to spontaneously occur.[47] So, as a result, when we say 'I am meditating' we actually mean 'I am creating the conditions in my mind that are conducive for dhyāna to occur.'[48]

It is important to note that these later limbs may not be accessible or helpful for students with mental health challenges, so it is important to go gently or even avoid speaking about them altogether until you and the student are ready.

GUṆAS

One of the main goals of yoga, and indeed of Mental Health Aware Yoga, is to increase sattva and to decrease rajas and tamas.

Sāṅkhya philosophy states that *Prakriti*, the material world, is made up of the three *guṇas*: *tamas*, *rajas* and *sattva*.[49] It is the interaction of the three guṇas that allows everything in the world (including the mind) to take on a unique characteristic.

Guṇas are thought to manifest in the following ways[50]:

SATTVA	RAJAS	TAMAS
Lucidity	Action	Inertia
Tranquillity	Hankering	Stillness
Wisdom	Attachment	Ignorance
Discrimination	Energetic endeavour	Delusion
Detachment	Passion	Disinterest
Happiness	Power	Lethargy
Peacefulness	Restlessness	Sleep
	Creative activity	Disinclination toward constructive activity

Guṇas can be both traits and states,[51] meaning that they can be a relatively constant attribute *and* also fluctuate throughout the day, depending on the circumstances. So, while you may generally be rajasic (trait), you may be become more tamasic after a long day at work and more sattvic after practising yoga (state).

From a mental health perspective, when we are feeling depressed, exhausted or hypo-aroused, finding it difficult to get out of bed and meet the day, *tamas* is likely to be predominant.

When we are feeling anxious, restless, agitated or hyper-aroused, finding it difficult to stay present and calm, the predominant guṇa is likely to be *rajas*.

And when we are experiencing positive mental health states, like happiness, wisdom and peacefulness, and are well within what Dr Daniel Siegel calls the Window of Tolerance,[52] then *sattva* is likely to be the predominant guṇa.

While sattva is considered to be the only quality of the mind that can lead to a reduction of *duḥkha* (suffering), there are times when tamas and rajas can be helpful.[53] If you want to go to sleep, it is going to be much easier if tamas is predominant. However, if you are wanting to teach a yoga class then an element of rajas is likely to be beneficial. Too much rajas could make the task difficult, but an element of rajas could help you to design and teach the class effectively. All three guṇas have necessary functions and it is important that we do not reject parts of ourselves in an effort to cultivate sattva.

The aim of the *yogi* (a serious practitioner of yoga) is to gain enlightenment or realization, and this is brought about by making sattva the dominant guṇa.[54] Hence, the practices of yoga are designed to reduce tamas and rajas and cultivate a predominance of sattva.[55] We will be exploring this in more depth in the Yogic Practices chapter.

COMPASSIONATE REFLECTION

1. Which guṇa is often predominant for you (trait)?
2. Right now, in this moment, which guṇa is dominant (state)?
3. What helps you to cultivate more sattva when you are feeling rajasic?
4. What helps you to cultivate more sattva when you are feeling tamasic?
5. What helps you to maintain your equilibrium when you are feeling sattvic?

KOSHAS

Koshas are *sheaths* or *layers* of our being, and represent different aspects of human existence, including the physical body, energy, emotions, thoughts and joy.

From gross to subtle, the koshas are:

1. *Annamaya* (physical body)
2. *Prāṇāmaya* (breath or the energetic body)
3. *Manomaya* (feeling and emotions)
4. *Vijnānamaya* (cognitions and the intellect)
5. *Ānāndamaya* (joy or bliss).

While we often think about mental illness as only affecting our emotions or thoughts, mental illness actually effects all the koshas.

When we are feeling depressed, we might feel heavy and lethargic in our body (annamaya); we may experience low energy, with restricted or shallow breathing (prāṇāmaya); we might feel sad or down (manomaya); have ruminative thoughts of hopelessness or helplessness (vijnānamaya) and feel disconnected from our innate state of joy or bliss (ānāndamaya).

When we are experiencing anxiety, we may be fidgety, hold tension in our jaw and have digestive issues (annamaya); we may have erratic energy with shallow and arrhythmic breathing patterns (prāṇāmaya); we may feel anxious or nervous (manomaya); have ruminative thoughts of not being good enough or worrying that something will go wrong (vijnānamaya) and feel disconnected from our innate state of joy (ānāndamaya).

This is why taking a holistic approach to mental health care is so important. When we focus on only one or two of the koshas, as we see in cognitive based psychotherapy or pharmacotherapy, we are not addressing the full spectrum of our being.

For yoga teachers who are not otherwise trained as mental health professionals or yoga therapists, I suggest focusing predominantly on annamaya and prāṇāmaya koshas by teaching āsana and prāṇāyāma. Doing so will naturally affect change on the other koshas and it also fits into a holistic model of mental health care, with yoga as an adjunct to other treatment modalities, such as psychotherapy, pharmacotherapy, nutrition and other lifestyle interventions.

Focusing on annamaya and prāṇāmaya can also help students to feel safe, inhabit their bodies and get out of the storm of thoughts and stories that often accompany mental health challenges and form the focus of psychotherapy. It also helps yoga teachers to stay within their scope of practice, so they can be confident that they are sharing safe and appropriate practices for the needs of their students, without causing harm.

Yoga teachers who are also mental health professionals or yoga therapists may consider widening their approach, drawing on their mental health training and clinical judgement to design a treatment protocol that integrates all five koshas.

COMPASSIONATE REFLECTION

1. When you are feeling rajasic, how does this affect the five koshas?
2. What about when you are feeling more tamasic?
3. Or sattvic?

Pillar Three

SAFE CONTAINER

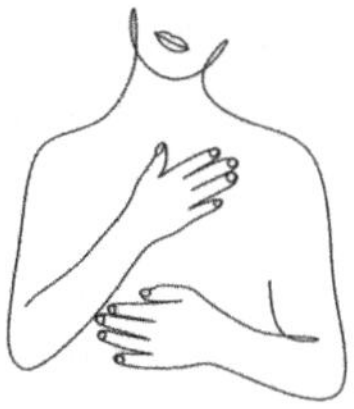

OVERVIEW

I believe that one of the best things we can do as yoga teachers, whether our students are experiencing mental health challenges or not, is to do what we can to create a safe and brave space where our students can come and connect with themselves, their fellow students, the teachings of yoga and us, as their teacher.

In this chapter, I outline some important ways that we might create a safe container, including the way we set up the environment, being present and predictable with our students, being mindful of touch and hands-on assists, supporting boundaries and self-care and being aware of ethical considerations.

While it is not actually possible to create a space that feels 100% safe and comfortable for everyone all of the time, there are some important things we can do to make this more likely, and we will be covering many of these in this chapter.

While I believe these suggestions for creating a safe container are important for everyone, they may be particularly important for students experiencing mental health challenges. So, if you are sharing yoga with students who you know are experiencing mental health challenges, or you are teaching in a setting where there is a reasonable chance of this (for example, in a mental health unit, a homeless support hub, an addiction recovery centre or with survivors of domestic violence), then I would suggest paying particular attention to safety and following as many of the suggestions in this chapter as you can.

THE ENVIRONMENT

Creating a safe container starts with the way we set up the space we teach in.

When setting up the room, take the time to really consider the effect that it will have on your students. When people walk into the Centre for Mind Body Wellness, a wellness centre I founded in Mullumbimby, Australia, many people who walk in say something like, 'Ahhh, it is so lovely and calm in here, I feel calmer just walking in.' This is an experience I consciously created with calming music, gentle lighting, beautiful but simple decor and an open and uncluttered space. It is like a little oasis in downtown Mullumbimby.

When you are setting up your teaching space, consider the niyama śauca and aim for an environment that is quiet, clean, uncluttered, private, relatively neutral, a comfortable temperature, has natural air flow and appropriate lighting and easy access to the bathroom and the exits. The environment is important when you are teaching online too. Pay attention to what is visible in the camera and aim for a calm and clean space.

While we do not always have control over the spaces we teach in, especially during home visits or when we are teaching in organizations or institutions, we can still understand the implications of the environment and do what we can to make it feel as safe and comfortable as possible.

Quiet

A quiet space is a joy for many people, but may be especially important for individuals with depression as they may have low serotonin levels, which can cause them to be more sensitive to sound.[1] I had a student in my class recently experiencing depression and anxiety, who said that he could not stand going to other yoga studios, as there was so much noise from the street that filtered in. He loved coming to my centre so much that he booked into the next course right after his course had finished.

It is not always possible to have a completely quiet space. The reality is that this can be very difficult; however, we can be mindful when selecting the spaces we teach in and aware of how sound might affect our students.

When teaching in spaces that are unavoidably noisy, like a home, a prison or a community or hospital setting, I suggest doing what you can to select a quieter space or quieter time of the day and, if possible, getting creative about how you might reduce the impact of the noise (for example, playing gentle music or white noise), and then surrendering the rest! The reality of life is that it can be noisy and busy and, for some people, it might actually be easier to practise within the hustle and bustle of life as it is less intimidating than a quiet space that feels unfamiliar and allows them to ruminate. For me personally, silence is bliss, but this is not true for everyone.

Students who have experienced trauma may be startled or triggered by loud noises outside the room. If this happens, it can be helpful to simply name the sound, for example, 'that sounds like a door slamming next door', and return to the practice.

When teaching online, it can be worth investing in a good quality microphone so students can hear your voice clearly and with less static and other noises from the room that you are teaching in.

Exits

People experiencing anxiety or those with a history of trauma may feel unsafe or unable to relax if they cannot easily access the exit or the bathroom.

You can help by ensuring that the bathroom is easily accessible and labelled so students know where to find it, and that exit doors are not locked on the inside during class so that people are free to come and go. It can also be helpful to ensure that students do not place their mats in front of the bathroom or exit doors, which can make it difficult to access them.

In some places, locking the door from the outside can help students to feel safe; however, be sure that students are not locked into the room that you are teaching in, as this can feel very unsafe.

Ideally, the exit and the bathroom doors are towards the back of the room, away from where you are standing and the direction that the students are facing, so that students can leave quietly without feeling observed by the whole class.

Privacy

As best you can, keep the teaching space private and out of view from the street or other rooms, so students do not feel observed by others outside the class. If you have any public-facing windows or glass doors, consider putting up curtains or a screen and, as best you can, organize it so classes are not interrupted by others, such as deliveries, other staff members or people walking through to access another part of the building.

If you are teaching online, inform your students in advance if you are recording the class and, if you are, let them know exactly what you are recording (e.g. just yourself or the whole class) and what you intend to do with the recording. Unless you have a clear reason (and consent) for recording your students, I would suggest only recording yourself, and not including your students in the recording at all.

Mirrors

As much as possible, avoid teaching in spaces with mirrors. If there are mirrors in the space you are teaching in (and this is becoming more and more popular in studios that also offer dance and pilates classes), consider covering them with fabric or a screen.

Having mirrors can communicate to students that the way we look when we practise yoga is important, whereas ideally we would like our students to pay more attention to the way yoga feels, rather than what it looks like.

Unfortunately, many people do not feel comfortable with the way they look, and having a mirror in the room can be difficult or triggering. Having mirrors also allows students to be seen from different angles, which could be uncomfortable for some students.

When teaching online, consider letting your students know that, if they wish, they can change their video settings so they only view the teacher, instead of watching themselves practise on the screen.

Lighting

Natural, soft light lighting can be ideal for a yoga space.

When lights are too bright, it can be glaring and uncomfortable, but if they are too dim it can feel unsafe and be triggering for some students. This can be true when teaching both in-person and online; however, for teaching online, professional soft lighting that illuminates you clearly can be helpful in supporting the students to easily see you and avoid confusion.

Emerson and Hopper suggest keeping the lights on and consistent throughout the class and not lowering the lights for Śavāsana at the end, as they found that doing so was disturbing for many of their students experiencing PTSD.[2]

While having the lights on in Śavāsana can be distracting for some students, consider offering your students an eye pillow to block out the light, then they can choose if they would like to use an eye pillow or not.

If you are teaching a candle-lit yoga class or a class that is intentionally held in a relatively dark space, be sure to communicate this clearly to your students in advance. This means that students can choose to attend or not based on their preference and comfort with dark places. For some students, a dark room could be a relief, as they are less likely to be seen, but for others it could be triggering and feel unsafe.

Smell

While some people enjoy incense and essential oils, others, especially highly sensitive people and those with chemical sensitivities or asthma, can find them intolerable. They may not be able to attend a class if there are strong scents or smells, or they may choose to come but leave with a headache or feeling unwell.

When I teach courses or workshops, I like to send an email to all the students beforehand, asking them to refrain from wearing scents or perfumes. This is because I know many of my students are sensitive to scents, but also because, while I can personally tolerate a small amount of natural scents, I often develop a headache if people around me are wearing synthetic fragrances or even essential oils.

Similarly, consider using natural and scent-free (or mild scent) cleaning products in the space you are teaching in and, unless your class is advertised as an essential oil class, avoid spraying your students with essential oil sprays. Even if you only spray essential oils on those students who consent to it, it is likely that the whole class will be able to smell it, and for someone who is sensitive to smells, it could still be overwhelming, even if it is not placed directly on their skin.

COMPASSIONATE REFLECTION

1. Which of these ideas are you already bringing into your teaching?
2. Were there any new ideas that you would like to bring into your classes?
3. Try out one of these ideas, then spend some time reflecting on how it went, including what went well, what did not go so well and what you would do differently next time.

BEING PRESENT

Giving your students your wholehearted and undivided attention, not just during the class but during the period before and after, can be such a gift.

It sounds simple, but it is easy to overlook.

Learning through experience

In the introduction, I shared about the very first adult yoga class that I ever taught. I was so nervous about leading the students through the sequence, and had carefully practised teaching the class many times beforehand. So, when I made it through the entire sequence and the students were lying quietly in Śavāsana, I was elated!

In my excitement, I left the students lying on their mats and went over to another intern teacher on the other side of the room and we quietly laughed, hugged and congratulated each other on a job well done.

That was until our mentor came over and told us in no uncertain terms that we were not to leave our students during Śavāsana, and we should definitely not be giggling and carrying on while they were still practising.

Ouch!

That deflated me immediately, but taught me a very important lesson about holding space that I have never forgotten.

Being present is not just about when your students are in Śavāsana, though. It begins from the moment your students come in the door to the moment they leave.

Being present during class

One very simple but very helpful way to be present when teaching yoga is to keep your eyes open at all times. If we are enjoying a practice that we are teaching, it can be tempting to close our eyes and focus on our own internal experience. However, it is important that we keep our eyes open at all times, observing and tracking our students so we can attend or respond to any questions, concerns or abreactions that might occur.

It can also feel very disconnecting for students if we spend time looking at our devices when teaching, so consider having your class plan on a piece of paper and, if you use music, preparing the play list in advance so you do not have to be looking at your device constantly during class.

Looking at a device while teaching can not only be disconnecting, it could also be triggering for some people who have experienced their friends or family being more interested in their devices than in them, or if they think that you are checking your emails or social media instead of wanting to be really present with them in the class, or if they are wondering if you going to take a photograph of them in class while they are not looking (the classic sneaky Śavāsana shot!).

Welcome and farewell your students

Being present and available when your students arrive and after the class can help to create a safe and welcoming container for your students.

I like to greet my students individually when they arrive and check in to see how they are doing or what they need in the class. And at the end of each class, I like to thank the group as a whole for attending and let them know that I am available for a few minutes afterwards to say 'hi' or check in. This can be done in a small group setting, but it also worth taking the extra time to do this even in a big studio class.

Checking in regularly in this way helps students know what to expect every time they come to your class; they know you will be present and available if they have something important to share with you before class or, if something challenging arises within the class, they know you will be available to chat for a short time with them afterwards.

Students will likely feel more able to trust in you and what you are teaching if they know you are present and available if they need support and to celebrate their achievements with them.

Be mindful that, while it can be helpful to be available for your students, you do need to be aware of your scope of practice and not take on the role of a therapist. If students start talking in detail about difficult experiences or past trauma, you might encourage them to speak with a mental health professional instead (more on this soon). It is also important to be respectful of your own time and energy and only stay chatting after class with students as long as feels comfortable to you (hello, boundaries!).

In summary, it can be helpful to your students when you are present, warm, available and approachable before, during and after class, while maintaining clear boundaries about your scope of practice and your time.

BEING PREDICTABLE

Attending a yoga class may be a huge endeavour for someone experiencing mental health challenges, and we can help them to feel safer and more comfortable by being predictable and not springing surprises on them.

Being predictable does not have to mean being boring. Instead, it can help students to feel safe and know what to expect.

There are many ways to be predictable for your students, including the way you set up the yoga space, welcoming and farewelling your students in a similar way each time, being clear in your class description about what you will be teaching, keeping the lights on all of the time, not moving around the room too much and letting students know how long they might stay in a posture or practice (of course inviting them to finish sooner or stay longer as they choose).

Be on time

Starting and ending your classes on time can help students to feel safe in your class, as they learn to trust that you will follow through with what you say you will do. It also respects and honours both your and your students' time.

Students experiencing mental health challenges may feel uncomfortable or anxious sitting around in the class waiting for you to start, and may show up just in time for the class to begin to avoid this. As a result, I suggest starting the class within a couple of minutes of the advertised start time, even if not everyone is there yet, and letting the students know that you respect their time, so will start the class on time as planned, but will welcome anyone who arrives late. This also creates a culture of punctuality and mutual respect, and students may be more likely to turn up on time as a result. It can also prepare students for the possibility of others coming in late, so they are less likely to be surprised or startled if this happens.

I have been to many classes where the teacher has run late, and I understand that this is likely to be coming from a place of generosity. However, for someone who is struggling, it may be taking all their resources just to stay until the end of the class and the extra 5–10 minutes might just feel too much. Or perhaps someone has organized child care, or needs to get back to work, and this means that they are running late for their other obligations and the class running late creates additional stress.

If you run over time, even on just one occasion, it may result in a student not returning to your class, or may mean that, in future classes, they cannot relax as they are keeping an eye on the time, as they cannot trust that you will finish at the time you said you would.

If you are coming towards the end of the class and realize that you are going to run late if you stick to your class plan, I suggest adapting your class plan and finishing on time, rather than pushing through and finishing late. Then, afterwards, consider reflecting on how you might plan your next class so you can finish on time.

TOUCH

Touch can be a contentious issue in the yoga world. It can be connecting and healing, but it can also be inappropriate, triggering and violating.

Inappropriate touch

One morning, I showed up to my regular pilates class and was surprised to find a male yoga teacher, whom I had never met, taking the place of our usual teacher. The class was given no notice that the usual teacher was away, the male yoga teacher was just there when we arrived.

Not long into the class, we were standing up on the reformer machines and sliding the platform in and out with our feet and trying to stay balanced. The teacher came up behind me and, in an attempt to correct my posture, ran his hands along the back side of my body, from my shoulders down to the back of my thighs.

He did not know me. I do not think he even knew my name. He did not ask if he could touch me or if I wanted his help. He just snuck up behind me and went ahead and placed his hands all over the back side of my body when I was in what felt like a very compromising position. If you have ever been on one of those reformer machines, I am sure you know what it is like to be balancing up there and just hoping that you do not fall off (or maybe that's just me?!).

Even though I am passionate about touch and consent in yoga and regularly teach on this topic, it still took a moment for me to find my voice and gather the courage to ask him to stop while the whole class was listening in.

He did take his hands off me after I clearly but politely asked him to, but he seemed very put out and told me that he did not know that I did not want to be touched. Unfortunately, defensiveness and shaming like this is very common when speaking up for yourself.

A few minutes later, we were lying on our backs on the reformer machine with our feet in the straps, moving our legs back-and-forth in a cycling motion.

Apparently, my technique was still not to his liking, as he picked up a wooden pilates stick, which was about 50cm long, and began touching me all over my body with the stick. He brandished it in front of the whole class like an old-fashioned school teacher about to cane a student and told everyone in the class that he was using the *naughty stick* on me.

Again, I asked him not to touch me.

He stopped touching me with his stick, but after a few minutes he picked up his iPad and began touching me with the device instead. At this time, I was still lying on the reformer machine on my back with my legs in straps in the air, feeling very vulnerable.

I was not the only one he touched in the class, but I was the only one who asked him not to. And after the first time I asked him, he only increased the touch, albeit with the *naughty stick* and his iPad, not his hands.

I probably should have walked out of the class, but I was there with my friend and I wanted to stay with her as she had just had a baby and I had not seen much of her lately. And, as much as I do not want to admit it, I did feel social pressure to smile and continue and not make a scene. This social conditioning can be strong!

I did, however, speak up several times during the class and contacted the owner of the studio later to let him know what had happened. He sent back a short message, apologizing and thanking me for my feedback and said that he would talk to the teacher. However, as far as I know, nothing changed, and I received no follow up, even when I attended classes later with the studio owner. I have since stopped going to this studio as a direct result of this incident.

Let me break down what felt inappropriate about this interaction for me:

- The teacher touched me without asking, in a position where I could not see him approaching.
- When I asked him to stop, he shamed me for doing so, in front of the whole class, implying it was my fault he did not know that I did not want to be touched.

- He continued to touch me with two different implements after I had asked him to stop.
- He implied I was being *naughty* for asking not to be touched by getting out the *naughty stick* and brandishing it like he was going to discipline me with it.
- He put on a show for the class at my expense, making a mockery of my discomfort.
- I did not know him and we had not established any rapport or trust that would indicate that his touch would be welcome.
- He was male. If a female teacher did the same, it still would not feel ok, but for me the sexual dynamic and the power imbalance would have been different.
- I was in a compromising position each time he touched me, first, balanced on the reformer machine and trying not to fall off, and, second, lying on my back with my legs held up in the air in straps, a position where I was not physically able to defend myself.
- A different teacher took the class without any notice, so I did not have the option to opt in or opt out of attending the class.
- The previous teacher, who was also male, had never touched anything more than my toes, and always in a way where I could anticipate it and it felt appropriate, so this kind of full body touch was not expected.
- As someone who has never experienced significant sexual trauma myself, I still hold the vicarious trauma of the millions of women in the world who have been sexually abused by men in positions of power, and the touch felt creepy, unsafe and inappropriate to me.

I have had several experiences like this and heard many similar stories from yoga students practising in all parts of the world; unfortunately, it is not an isolated incident.

Alternatives to touch

Touch, or hands-on assists, are not the only way to guide your students if they need support or direction in class. Both *verbal* and *visual* cues can clearly and effectively communicate your message without ever touching your students.

Verbal assisting is when you speak (rather than touch) to communicate with your students. Just like we can guide our students through a yoga practice with our words alone, we can also offer guidance for adapting or adjusting the practice, using our words. It takes skill and practice to refine our language to offer verbal assists but, with practice, it can become a highly effective and caring way to support our students.

Visual assisting is where the teacher demonstrates on themselves, in view of the student. Just like we can demonstrate in a yoga class by doing the practices ourselves, we can also demonstrate an adjustment or a refinement that we would like to offer the student. For example, if a student is in Vīrabhadrāsana (Warrior Pose), and their front knee looks like it might be in an uncomfortable position, we may come into a Vīrabhadrāsana (Warrior Pose) ourselves, place a hand on our own knee, and demonstrate moving the knee gently into a position that may be more comfortable and supportive.

By using verbal or visual assists, or a combination of both, you not only guide the student with their practice but you also communicate your respect for the student's personal boundaries and your care and interest in them. Some students may never have experienced this respect and care, and it can be profound for the student and helpful in cultivating a secure and healthy relationship between the student and teacher.

And when we drop the need for practices to look a certain way, or to get it *right*, there is less and less need to offer our students assists or refinements at all.

Hands-on assists

So does this mean that we should never touch our students?

Not necessarily.

It does mean that we need to respect our students' boundaries and be conscious whether or not to use touch in our yoga classes. We need to ask ourselves if touch could be triggering for the student, if it is taking the student towards or away from their internal experience and if it is *actually* necessary.

If you are sharing yoga with students who you know have experienced trauma, or you are teaching in a setting where there is a reasonable chance that the students coming to your class may have a lived experience of trauma (e.g. a community setting, a mental health unit, a homeless support hub, an addiction recovery centre or with survivors of domestic violence), then I would suggest that you avoid touching your students completely and instead rely solely on verbal and visual cues.

Even if you are sharing yoga with students in a setting where you feel that touch would be beneficial, remember that you can never know for sure if someone has experienced trauma, so always be mindful when offering touch, and consider initially offering verbal or visual cues before offering hands-on assists.

If you do discern that hands-on assists may be helpful in your class, an easy and important rule of thumb is to not offer touch to students you do not know well. It takes time to establish trust and to get to know a student enough to ascertain if touch might be appropriate and helpful. I suggest waiting until you have developed a relationship with a student before offering touch.

If you do believe touch to be the most appropriate way to support your student, always (always) ask. Consent is paramount. Never touch a student without first asking them, even if you have touched them many times before.

When offering a hands-on assist, consider standing where the student can clearly see you, making eye contact, and clearly explain the touch that you are offering. Remember that just because a student consented to touch in the past, it does not mean that they consent to touch all of the time. A student may appreciate hands-on assists in some practices but not others, or by some teachers but not others, or on some days of their menstrual cycle but not others. So, always ask.

I have heard some teachers say that they just intuitively know if a student wants to be touched or not, so they do not need to ask.

To be blunt, this is naive at best and abusive at worst.

Granted, we could sense if a student would appreciate hands-on assists or not. But we cannot know for certain and it is arrogant to presume that we do. So, always ask.

Even when asked, students may consent to touch even though they do not really want it, so it is important to always communicate with your words *and* your body language that it is completely acceptable (and indeed encouraged) to say *no*. Students will be noticing your interactions with other students in the class, so for students to feel safe to say *no*, they need to see you genuinely communicating and honouring choice with *all* your students.

This discrepancy between the student's communicated consent and their actual needs can happen because of the power imbalance between the teacher and the student. The student may wish to please us, feel embarrassed to say *no* or feel like there will be consequences if they refuse. They might believe that we know their body and what they need better than they do. We can reinforce this belief and, in doing so, disempower the student if we are not mindful in the way we offer touch. The student may have had the experience in previous classes, or in other parts of their life, where their choices around touch were not honoured and feel powerless to assert their needs. The student may also want to conform, want us to like them, or to be a *good student* and, as a result, consent to touch, even though they do not actually want it or feel comfortable with it.

If touch or hands-on assists are an important feature of your teaching style, consider including this in the class description. This means that students can make an informed decision to attend your class or not in advance, rather than finding themselves in an awkward position where they are one of the only students in the class who are saying *no* to your touch.

Consent Tokens

One simple and effective way to begin conversations about touch and consent, and for students to communicate their preferences about touch, is to use Consent Tokens or something similar.

The Consent Tokens that we have created at Mental Health Aware Yoga have the word *yes* on one side and the word *no* on the other, so students can quickly, easily and subtly communicate their preferences, not just at the beginning of class but at any time throughout.

It is not enough to simply place the Consent Tokens at the front door and ask students to take them if they would like, or even to place a Consent Token on each students' mat with the *yes* side facing up.

The best practice for using Consent Tokens includes placing a token on every student's mat at the beginning of class with the *no* side facing up, inviting them to change it to *yes* if they would like hands-on assists, and letting them know they can change the Consent Token at any time during class.

By placing the Consent Tokens on the mats with the *no* side facing up, your students have to actively choose to say *yes*, rather than it being the default. They need to opt-*in* to touch, rather than opt-*out* of it.

This is a mistake that I see many yoga teachers make when they ask their students to raise their hand at the beginning of class if they do not want to be touched, even if all the students are in Balāsana (Child's Pose) and it is less likely that others will see their preference. It can be difficult to speak up or raise your hand to say that you do not wish to be touched, so it is important that *no* touch is the default.

Doing so means that your students are more likely to choose *yes* when they actually mean *yes*, rather than consent because they feel pressured or embarrassed to say *no*.

If you are teaching in a yoga studio, I suggest introducing the Consent Tokens to all of the classes, so students come to expect them and are more likely to feel safe in every class they attend.

Even when a student indicates with their Consent Token that they are open to hands-on assists, I suggest always asking before touching them anyway. While they may generally be open to touch, they may not wish to be touched in a particular practice or in a particular way.

Always ask (have I said that enough yet?).

Empowerment and choice

As we saw in the Western Psychology chapter, what makes an experience traumatic is often the feeling of powerlessness that we had during the experience. And, when we are feeling depressed or anxious, we can often feel helpless, hopeless and powerless about our circumstances.

As yoga teachers, offering our students choice about touch and hands-on assists, and deeply honouring the choices they make, has the potential to be a healing experience, increasing self-agency and self-empowerment. On the flip side, when we do not offer and honour choice, we can reinforce this experience of powerlessness.

The way I see it, offering hands-on assists is *less* about the hands-on assists themselves and *more* about the conversations that we have about consent and body autonomy, the opportunities for students to enquire into their own needs and the deep respect we show for our students by asking what they want and honouring these needs. This has the potential to be healing and life changing, and goes far beyond the benefits that a student might receive from the physical act of touch or a hands-on assist.

Appropriate touch

If you decide that touch is the best way to support your student, and they have clearly consented to it, there are some important things to consider.

First of all, ensure that you are properly educated and skilled in offering hands-on assists and have an understanding of the potential psychological and physical pitfalls. Hands-on assists require extensive training, practice and sensitivity, so make sure that you have all of these before touching your students.

Check in with yourself to ensure that the touch is for your student's benefit only, not for yours. Ask yourself if the hands-on assist is because you would like the practice to look a certain way, or if it is actually beneficial for the student, and if a hands-on assist would be taking the student towards or away from their own internal experience.

Be mindful of how and where you touch your students. As a guide, I suggest not touching your students' genitals, bottom or breasts and not touching your genitals, bottom or breasts against your students' body or positioning them in front of their face. Keep the touch as minimal as possible, and do not linger. Keep your sexual energy in check and do not bring it into the yoga room nor into a hands-on assist.

If a student tells you they would like a hands-on assist, but during the assist lets you know that they have changed their mind or if something in their body language suggests that they are not comfortable with it, stop touching your student immediately; thank them for letting you know, apologize if necessary and be careful not to shame them or make them feel wrong about changing their mind or not wanting what you are offering. Remember, it is not about you. Your students knowing what is best for them and their body and being able to communicate it, is something to be celebrated, not dismissed or shamed.

As I write this, I keep pausing to put my head in my hands, dismayed that this bears mentioning at all. But given the repeated allegations of inappropriate touch and sexual abuse happening in yoga circles, and my own experience being touched by yoga teachers, it seems like it does. There is still a lot of work to do around touch and consent in yoga, so I am so glad that you are here reading this book and being part of this new paradigm. It is time!

COMPASSIONATE REFLECTION

1. What has been your experience of receiving touch or hands-on assists as a yoga student?
2. What has been your journey with providing touch or hands-on assists as a teacher?
3. Has anything changed after reading this section on touch and consent?
4. What would you like to do differently?

BOUNDARIES

On the whole, I have found that yoga teachers are often not the best at setting and maintaining personal boundaries. Yoga teachers tend to be generous and caring souls and want to go above and beyond for their yoga students, often at the expense of their own wellbeing. Sound familiar?

However, when we do not set and maintain clear boundaries, we are likely headed for burnout or compassion fatigue, and that is not good for us, nor for our students. So, for your own wellbeing, and the wellbeing of your students, having clear and compassionate boundaries is vital.

As a reforming chronic people pleaser, having clear boundaries has been a challenging journey for me. What I have found, though, from my own experience and from working with many clients around this issue, is that when we do not set or when we have unclear boundaries, or when we are not prepared to defend our boundaries when necessary, people will be confused about what is okay and what is not okay for us, and will either intentionally or unintentionally cross our boundaries over and over again. And that gets exhausting!

Instead of feeling resentful, which is what often arises when people repeatedly cross our boundaries, we need to take responsibility for clearly communicating our boundaries in advance and defending them, if necessary, even if it feels uncomfortable. If you are not sure what your boundaries are, simply consider what feels okay for you and what does not.

Do you feel okay spending 30 minutes chatting to students about their yoga practice after class, or would five minutes feel better? If the latter is true, consider letting your students know at the end of class that you will be around for five minutes afterwards and are available for questions, and be sure to wrap up the discussion after five minutes, so you are true to your word.

Do you feel okay with students cancelling a private session ten minutes before the scheduled appointment, or would 24 hours' notice feel better? Whatever your preference is, a written consent form that clearly states your cancellation policy can be helpful to clarify your terms and conditions, and make sure that you follow through with them if students do cancel.

Do you feel okay with a student calling you at the weekend, or do you want to keep your weekends for personal time and need a separate work phone that you can turn off on weekends and evenings?

Are you prepared to enforce these boundaries if a student crosses them?

While it can be initially uncomfortable, I find that the easiest way to have clear boundaries is to be upfront about them and, for the most part, I have found that people are very understanding, and often inspired, when the terms and conditions of working with me are clear.

COMPASSIONATE REFLECTION

1. What are your personal boundaries in regard to your yoga teaching?
2. How might you communicate them in advance with your students?
3. How might you uphold these boundaries if a student or colleague crosses them?

SELF-PRACTICE, SELF-CARE AND SELF-ENQUIRY

Yoga therapist and teacher trainer Saraswathi Vasudevan says that the *state* of the yoga teacher is 95% of the transmission of yoga and knowledge is only 5%.[3] So it is less about *what* we teach and more about *how* we show up when we teach yoga.

To show up fully for our students, it is important to have established ourselves in practices of self-care, self-practice and self-enquiry.

For me, self-care means, as best I can, tuning into my needs on a moment-by-moment basis and being willing to meet them. It sounds simple, but living in the busy and sometimes overwhelming world that we live in where self-care is often seen as selfish or a last-minute concern, it is not always easy. But it is very important for mental health.

Self-care does not have to mean massages and manicures. It might look like going to bed early when you are tired, meditating in the morning, spending time by yourself when you are feeling overwhelmed, spending time with friends when you feel like company, spending time in nature, walking the dog, taking holidays and getting support with your mental health when you need it.

There is no one-size-fits-all prescription for self-care. Self-care is anything that feels nourishing and life enhancing to you.

As Mental Health Aware Yoga teachers, an important part of self-care is having a regular yoga practice of our own. Having our own practice is important for our own mental health, so that we can hold space for our students in a way that is really present, balanced and nourishing and so we can show up for our students authentically steeped in the wisdom and practice of yoga.

The challenges you face with your own practice will also help you to understand the challenges your students face. When I was teaching a lot of yoga classes (at one point it was around 16 classes per week) I had the experience, like so many yoga teachers do, of letting my own yoga practice fall by the wayside. But teaching is not the same as self-practice. When we are teaching, we are holding space for our students, and when we are practising, we are holding space for ourselves. Having our own personal practice is important. There is no way around it. And I am writing this now for myself as much as I am writing it for you! I know it is not always easy, so go gently on yourself, but keep coming back to your practice (this is the tension between svādhyāya and tapas we explored in the Yoga Psychology chapter).

Another important part of a personal practice is self-enquiry. This can be any type of yoga or meditation that focusses on self-enquiry, or even journalling or psychotherapy if you choose. Being willing to enquire compassionately, non-judgementally and honestly into our own nature, is, I believe, an essential part of being a wise and compassionate yoga teacher.

While I have only briefly touched on these elements of self-practice, self-care and self-enquiry, it does not mean that they are not important. We could spend a lifetime exploring these, and I hope that you do.

COMPASSIONATE REFLECTION

1. On a scale from one to ten, how would you rate your own self-care?
2. Is there anything you would like to do differently? If so, what is it?

3. What is your personal yoga practice?
4. Is there anything you would like to do differently? If so, what is it?
5. What is your personal practice of self-enquiry?
6. Is there anything you would like to do differently? If so, what is it?

HELPING (NOT RESCUING)

I imagine that part of the reason you are a yoga teacher, and are reading this book, is because you want to help people. I do too.

However, it is vital that we do not fall into the trap of believing that we are saving, rescuing or fixing anybody.

When we try to rescue people from their own lives and their own problems, we risk burnout for ourselves and disempowerment for others.

When we take the role of the rescuer, even if it is not conscious, we cast the other person in the role of the helpless victim, and essentially communicate to them that we know better and that we do not believe that they have what it takes to solve their own problems.

As Mental Health Aware Yoga teachers, it is *not* our role to fix our students' problems, nor to take responsibility for our students' choices or situations.

However, it *is* our role to teach yoga in a way that cultivates sattva, to create a relatively safe container to teach in, to listen compassionately to our students and to do what we can to empower them to trust in their own wholeness and intuition and, based on this, make decisions for themselves.

You might notice that you have slipped into the role of rescuer if you find yourself telling your students what do to with their lives, if you are lying awake at night thinking about your students' problems, if you are feeling resentful that a student is not taking your advice, if you are feeling like you need to have the answer to everything, if you are trying to stop students from crying or if you are doing things for your students they could be doing for themselves (or that their friends, family or therapist could be doing for them).

If you notice any of these signs, consider talking to your mentor or therapist about what is happening and reconnect with your role as a teacher.

COMPASSIONATE REFLECTION

1. Do you remember a time when someone tried to fix or rescue you? How did it make you feel?
2. Do you have a tendency to try to rescue or save your students? If so, what do you tend to do?
3. What changes would you like to make in your own life to stop trying to fix or rescue others?

SCOPE OF PRACTICE

To teach within your scope of practice means to only teach within your area of expertise.

As a trained yoga teacher, your scope of practice is to work within the specialized skills and knowledge of a yoga teacher. If you have other qualifications and experience, for example as a psychologist, counsellor, naturopath, physiotherapist, doctor, yoga therapist or ayurvedic practitioner, then your scope of practice will be extended accordingly.

Unless you are qualified in another area, your scope of practice as a yoga teacher does not include offering counselling, medical advice, relationship advice, nutrition advice, life coaching, ayurvedic treatments, yoga therapy, aromatherapy or herbal supplements.

Yoga Australia, a yoga teachers association in Australia that I am a member of, describes the role of the yoga teacher as working within an educational framework.[4]

They describe the scope of practice for yoga teachers as:

- Working within the scope of a yoga teaching qualification with a variety of physical, emotional, mental and spiritual health presentations.
- Offering an integrated set of practices aligned to the needs of the individual and according to yogic models of health, including (but not limited to) the koshas and guṇas.
- Teaching yoga practices such as āsana, prāṇāyāma, relaxation, meditation, mudra, bandha, mantra, bhavana (imagery) and sankalpa (intention).
- Sharing information on yoga philosophy and yogic lifestyle.
- Working in a group class consisting of people with a variety of conditions (with individual assessment provided prior to entry to the class and individual modifications given) and individualized yoga teaching in one-to-one settings.

As yoga teachers, we can be so good at creating a safe space that our students often confide in us and ask us for advice in various areas of their lives. But we need to be mindful that we do not know everything, and in fact we do not have to know everything. For me, personally, that feels like a huge relief!

COMPASSIONATE REFLECTION

1. What is your personal scope of practice?
2. Is there anything you would like to change about your teaching or the way you support your students after reflecting on your scope of practice?

CLOTHING

A primary school principal once told me the rule she had for the teacher's dress code at her school. She said: 'If you can see up it, down or through it, don't wear it.' I believe that this a good rule of thumb for yoga teachers too.

However, teaching yoga is clearly different to primary school teaching, and in some situations it might be appropriate for teachers to wear more revealing clothing, for example, if it is necessary for students to see a part of the teacher's body in a particular posture or practice.

But when the teacher's clothing is sexualized, focused on exhibiting the body or overly branded, then it may detract from the teaching. I believe that it is the teacher's job to create a safe and sacred space for the teachings to be shared, and, by dressing modestly and in a way that does not distract from the teachings, we can support our students to focus on their own practice and the teachings that we are sharing.

This is not about being a prude or about denying our sexuality, but about recognizing our role as a teacher and being clear about our intentions when we dress for class. Students notice what we wear and, like it or not, it is part of the message that we are sharing when we stand in front of our students.

So, where do we draw the line between what is appropriate and what is not? What is a healthy appreciation for the body and the wonderful things it can do, versus being over-sexualized, over-exhibiting and detracting from the teachings of yoga? I do not have all the answers, but I am definitely interested in exploring the questions, and I hope you are too.

COMPASSIONATE REFLECTION

1. How do you dress when teaching yoga?
2. Do you feel that it is appropriate for teaching yoga, or does it detract from your teaching in some way?
3. Is there anything you would like to do differently?

SOCIAL MEDIA AND PROMOTION

Promoting yoga classes and offerings, whether it is on social media, on your website or on a printed flyer, can be an effective way for yoga teachers to share their love of yoga and promote their classes. However, many yoga teachers I know have a complicated relationship with social media and promotion.

History of yoga promotion

Taking photographs in impressive postures to promote yoga is not new. In the book *Krishnamacharaya: His Life and Teachings*, Krishnamacharaya's long-time student A. G. Mohan writes about how Krishnamacharaya would have his daughter, Shubha, demonstrate difficult yoga postures and have photographs taken of himself in intense yoga postures with the clear intention of popularizing yoga.[5]

When A. G. Mohan asked Krishnamacharaya how a yoga teacher could teach these intense āsanas to ordinary people with health issues, Krishnamacharaya replied: 'It was a demonstration for propaganda! You should not take it literally. Shubha can do it, but for the others you must suggest appropriate asanas. Only the principle is important.'[6]

If you see photographs of Krishnamacharya in these promotional photographs, he does not wear much in the way of clothes, his chest and his legs are bare, and he demonstrates some pretty difficult postures. What he did not do (as far as I am aware) was share photographs of himself that were naked, sexualized or body image focused. As far as I am aware, these photos were to demonstrate the postures in order to encourage people to try yoga, not to exhibit his body.

Social media and yoga teachers

Yoga teachers seem to be divided on the use of social media and promotion. Some see it as a necessary evil and use it in order to promote their classes, others see it as a wonderful way to share the message of yoga and promote their work and others shy away from it altogether, seeing it as selling out. I believe that this is a decision that each of us must make for ourselves.

However, if you do choose to use social media, I suggest keeping the yamas and niyamas in mind and adding to the conversation in a way that is authentic and empowering for those who choose to follow you, rather than leaving people feeling not good enough about themselves and disenchanted with yoga.

COMPASSIONATE REFLECTION

1. What are your thoughts on promoting your yoga classes on social media?
2. If you are sharing about yoga on social media, what are you doing to share in way that is authentic and empowering?
3. Is there anything you would like to change?

SEXUAL RELATIONSHIPS WITH STUDENTS

In a yoga shala I practised in in Mysuru, India, in my twenties, there was a sign that read, 'no romancing in the Shala.' My then boyfriend (now husband) and I giggled at it at the time, but it is an important point about the student–teacher relationship that is often not talked about until it is too late.

As we explored in the brahmacarya section of the Yoga Psychology chapter, it is important that we do not bring our sexual energy into the student–teacher relationship and do not engage in sexual relationships with our students.

No sexual relationships with students

Psychologists, and many other registered health professionals, are not permitted to engage in any sexual activity with current or previous clients, and risk being deregistered (and therefore unable to work in the profession) or face legal action if they do.

While yoga teachers are encouraged to conduct themselves in accordance with the yamas and niyamas, there are no clear ethical standards regarding sexual engagement with students, and no real consequences for yoga teachers if they do.

To keep the student–teacher relationship safe and to hold the teachings of yoga sacred, I recommend that yoga teachers do not engage in any sexual activities or relationships with their students.

There is a natural imbalance of power in the student–teacher relationship, and a student may feel that they are not able to say *no* to the advances of their yoga teacher, as they fear the possibility of losing their teacher, their sanctuary, their practice and their community. Other students in the class may feel uncomfortable witnessing a yoga teacher making advances on another student or developing a new romantic relationship, and they may no longer see the class as a safe space.

As a student, it can be seductive to have someone be endlessly present, kind, compassionate and encouraging, the way a yoga teacher often is. So, it is not uncommon for a student to develop romantic feelings for a teacher and imagine that the teacher would be an ideal romantic partner or lover.

However, while the teacher may be adept at holding space during the class, outside of class and in relationships, they likely have the same foibles and relationship challenges as everyone else that the student is not necessarily privy to. As a result, the student may have an unrealistic idea of what a relationship with their teacher would be like.

It is the responsibility of the teacher, not the student, to understand the intricate dynamics of the student–teacher relationship and to avoid engaging in sexual activities or romantic relationships.

Managing sexual attraction to a student

Yoga teachers have sexual and relationship needs the same as everyone else. However, it is important that, as teachers, we get our social, emotional and sexual needs met outside the student–teacher relationship and consciously cultivate romantic relationships or circles of friends and family to meet these needs.

Feeling a sexual attraction to a student is normal, but it is your responsibility as the teacher not to act on it.

If you do experience a sexual attraction to a student, I suggest noticing the attraction arising within you, spending some time afterwards enquiring into it and speaking to your mentor, therapist or an experienced and compassionate peer openly about it.

Your enquiry might include:

- How do I experience this in my body?
- What thoughts and emotions are present?
- What actions or urges are arising?
- What is it about this student that I am attracted to?
- If I acted on this attraction, what needs of mine would be met?
- How else could I meet these needs (either by myself or with another)?
- If I acted on this attraction, what could the pitfalls be for me?
- If I acted on this attraction, what could the pitfalls be for the student?
- What is the best interest of the student?
- If I were mentoring another yoga teacher in a similar situation, what advice would I give them?

If the attraction continues after this process of self-enquiry, consider ending the student–teacher relationship with the student, so the student can continue to practise yoga without the interference of your attraction.

If the attraction continues and is mutual, after consulting with your mentor, therapist or an experienced peer, consider having an open conversation with your student about your feelings and about the ethical dilemma of sexual relationships with students. It may be necessary to end the student–teacher relationship, as it is not appropriate for a yoga teacher to be in a sexual or romantic relationship while the student–teacher relationship is still current.

COMPASSIONATE REFLECTION

1. Has a student ever been attracted to you? How did you handle it?
2. Have you ever been attracted to a student? What did you do?
3. If the answer was yes to either of these questions, do you have a compassionate and non-judgemental mentor or therapist you could explore this with?

SPEAKING UP

So, what do we do if we believe a yoga teacher is behaving inappropriately with a student? Do we just keep quiet in the belief that it is none of our business, or do we say something and risk speaking out?

In many countries registered health professionals have a legal obligation to notify the health regulation body if another health professional is behaving unethically.

As far as I am aware, yoga teachers have no such mandatory reporting; however, I believe that we should adhere voluntarily to the same standards.

Unfortunately, there are far too many examples of yoga teachers behaving inappropriately. As yoga teachers, I believe that it is important to not only behave ethically ourselves, but be willing to stand up and speak out when other yoga teachers are not.

If you believe that another yoga teacher has behaved unethically and inappropriately, I suggest discussing it with your mentor and, if it feels safe and appropriate, to speak directly to the yoga teacher in question to address it with them. If the inappropriate behaviour is happening with an individual student, consider speaking to them and asking what you can do to help. Beware of stepping into the role of the rescuer!

If the inappropriate behaviour is serious (for example, sexual abuse or causing harm) or the teacher continues the behaviour after your discussion, you might consider contacting your national yoga teachers' association, the police or other relevant authority.

It can be difficult to speak up against a member of your own yoga teaching community; however, it is arguably an important part of living your yoga, including ahiṁsā, satya, asteya and brahmacarya.

COMPASSIONATE REFLECTION

1. Have you ever witnessed, or known of, an abusive yoga teacher? If so, what did you do?
2. Would you do anything differently now?
3. Do you know of any inappropriate behaviour from a yoga teacher that is occurring now? If so, what will you do about it?

MENTORING

Mentoring is traditionally how yoga was passed from teacher to student, with teachers handing down information to students on a one-to-one basis over an extended period of time. It was also how yoga students would eventually become teachers.

With the rise of teacher training programs and national standards in education to become a registered yoga teacher, this has changed significantly.

While nowadays the initial training for yoga teachers is most often a 200-hour programme taken over a relatively short period of time, usually from one month to one year, I believe that it is important that yoga teachers continue to engage in ongoing mentoring.

Mentoring is important for:

- the ongoing growth of competent, compassionate and skilful teachers
- self-enquiry and self-reflection
- addressing gaps and developing knowledge, skills and education
- compassionately and non-judgementally exploring ethical dilemmas

- accountability with self-practice and self-care
- creating community, instead of teaching and practising in isolation.

Ideally, mentoring would include a combination of:

- regular one-to-one mentoring sessions with a senior yoga teacher or specialist in the area you are working in
- regular peer-to-peer mentoring with another yoga teacher, offering each other support
- ongoing training
- group mentoring sessions with a senior yoga teacher or specialist in the area you are working in.

In the Mental Health Aware Yoga training, we offer all graduates the option to join our Mental Health Aware Yoga Teachers' Community, to continue with professional development and group mentoring long after the training has finished.

COMPASSIONATE REFLECTION

1. What has been your experience of mentoring in the past?
2. What gaps in your mentoring would you like to address?

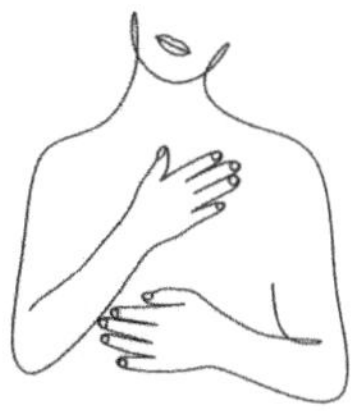

Pillar Four

THERAPEUTIC SKILLS

While yoga teachers are not therapists (unless of course, otherwise qualified), there are some very helpful therapeutic skills that yoga teachers can bring into their teaching to support their students' mental health.

In this chapter, I am going to share some of these, including meeting your students where they are, encouraging an individualized practice, sharing interpersonal and intrapersonal rhythms, using skilful language and fostering embodiment.

MEET THEM WHERE THEY ARE

One of the most delightful things we can do for our students is to *meet them where they are.*

This includes both *accepting* our students as they are and *sequencing* a class that builds from where they are into a more sattvic state.

Acceptance

Many people start practising yoga as they want to change something about themselves. They want to be thinner, stronger, more flexible, less stressed, anxious or depressed or have more friends.

All of these can come from practising yoga, and we know that change happens as a result of a dedicated yoga practice; however, it is important as Mental Health Aware Yoga teachers that we fully see and accept our students just as they are, not just focused on the changes that they want to make.

This act of genuine acceptance is a remarkable gift, one that is surprisingly rare and holds immense potential for connection and healing.

When we recognize our students' inherent perfection and divine spark, not just as a nice idea or philosophy, but fully and deeply see them in their unique wholeness and perfection, we offer them something very special and possibly something very different to their other experiences in the world.

We are all constantly bombarded with messages that we need to be something other than who we are. Advertising is built on the premise of finding people's *pain points* and offering them a solution that will change this (i.e. a product or service). Even therapy is largely built on the idea that something is dysfunctional or disordered and needs an expert to *fix* it.

As humans, and particularly as yoga teachers, I believe that we need to be able to hold the paradox of being perfect just as we are with the somewhat conflicting desire for growth and ongoing development. Both can be true. We can be inherently whole and perfect and at the same time seek growth and change. And when we do this, we grow and change from a place of wholeness, not from a place of brokenness. There is a world of difference.

Class sequencing

When we offer sequences to our students to assist them to move from a more rajasic or tamasic state to a more sattvic state, the best place to start is most often where the student already is.

If a student has a predominance of rajas, then generally the best place to start is with more rajasic or active practices. If they have a predominance of tamas, ideally, we would start with more tamasic or nourishing practices. Sounds counterintuitive, right?

While active practices like Sūrya Namaskar (Sun Salutation) can be up-regulating and help to reduce tamas, if you ask someone with tamasic depression to start their yoga practice with dynamic Sūrya Namaskars, they may find it very difficult to get started and may not want to practise.

Similarly, while nourishing practices like a long supported Śavāsana (Corpse Pose) can be down-regulating and help to reduce rajas, if you ask someone with a rajasic anxiety to start their practice in this way, they will likely find it very difficult and may give up or not come back to your class ever again.

Instead, we can make yoga more accessible and keep our students engaged by meeting them where they are and supporting them, over the duration of the class, to gradually shift to a more sattvic state.

So, for a class of students who are predominately rajasic, you might start with a dynamic Sūrya Namaskar practice and gradually slow the class down and finish in a supported Śavāsana.

For a class that is predominately tamasic, you might start in supported Balāsana (Child's Pose) or another gentle posture and gradually make the class more and more active, inviting the students to try Sūrya Namaskars towards the end of the class.

This, of course, is easier to do a private class with only one student, but it is possible in group classes too. We will explore this more in the Yogic Practices chapter.

INDIVIDUALIZED PRACTICE

Yoga is not a performance sport. Unlike ballet, where the focus is on what the body *looks* like and the emphasis is often on the dancers moving identically and in synchronization, the focus of yoga is more about what it *feels* like and what the individual *needs* in each moment.

While it may look impressive for a group of students to be moving gracefully together, in our yoga classes, it is more important that our students make choices based on their own needs and find their own individualized practice within the class.

I have heard yoga teachers complain about their students doing different variations or different postures than what they were teaching in class; however, I believe that this is something to be celebrated, not frowned upon. As a yoga teacher, I feel like I am doing a great job if I see my students practising in a way that is right for them, rather than trying to be a *good student* and follow my instructions to the letter.

We can create an environment for an individualized practice to occur, in either a group or one-on-one setting, by offering choices and encouraging students to practise in a way that feels right for them.

Choice and mental health

Individuals experiencing depression, anxiety or trauma may feel a sense of hopelessness and helplessness, lack self-efficacy and feel like there is very little that they can do to change their circumstances.

By inviting our students to *choose* a way to practise that works for them, we can provide a space to reclaim a sense of autonomy and self-efficacy. This can be a subtle but profoundly beneficial part of their healing journey.

Introducing choice into your teaching

When teaching, try offering your students a few different variations of each posture or sequence. This can make it more accessible to students and can also encourage your students to practise in a way that is most in alignment with their needs and intention for their practice. You could try offering suggestions for different arm positions, or a standing versus seated version of the practice or a more dynamic versus nourishing variation.

Too many choices may be confusing, especially for folk who find decision making challenging or those who are new to yoga. However, offering a couple of variations, as well as the option to rest in Balāsana (Child's Pose) or any other comfortable position at any time, can be a great way to empower your students to check in with their own needs and practise in a way that feels best for them.

Be mindful, however, of the way you offer choice and the language that you use when you do.

Often teachers will offer choice, but present it in a way that makes one variation seem better than the other. For example, a teacher might share a practice like Vṛkṣāsana (Tree Pose) and instruct their students to rest the sole of the foot high on their inner thigh, and then let their students know that, if they cannot balance very well or are not strong enough, they can rest their toes on the floor or lean against the wall for support.

While this is offering choice, it is also communicating to the student that there is a *correct* way to do the practice and the variations are only available if you are not *good enough* to do it the *right* way.

Instead, you could offer different *variations* (instead of different *levels*), including the toes resting on the floor, or placing the sole of the foot at any height along the standing leg that feels comfortable; of course, there is always the option to create more stability by placing a hand on the wall. As a teacher, after demonstrating possible variations, consider doing the most accessible version yourself. Modelling this can empower students to see the value in responding to their bodies' needs rather than feeling they need to push themselves to do a variation that is difficult for them.

Instead of using words like *modifications*, *easier and harder versions* or the *correct version*, try offering different *options* or *variations* of the practice, or describe different ways to practise based on whether the student is seeking an *activating* practice or a *nourishing* practice. This language can direct students to their internal experience and support them to make a choice based on their needs or intentions in the moment, not on getting it *right*.

And, finally, when offering choice, try encouraging your students to move towards comfort, rather than discomfort. This simple cue can revolutionize the way we practice and teach yoga.

We will go into more detail about language later in this chapter.

Offer Balāsana

I like to encourage my students to listen to their bodies and rest or pause whenever needed. This might mean resting in Balāsana (Child's Pose), or perhaps Tadāsana (Mountain Pose), Śavāsana (Corpse Pose) or Constructive Rest, depending on what feels the most comfortable and nourishing for the student. I have found that while many people love Balāsana, others find it uncomfortable, so be willing to vary the posture for some students or offer other shapes instead.

I have heard about students who spent the majority of a class in Balāsana or Śavāsana, and when the teacher checked in with them afterwards, they said they loved the class, and just being in the room, doing a few practices and listening to the teacher was a wonderful experience. Just because it may not look like a student is fully engaged in the class, it does not mean that they are not getting something from the experience. It may be exactly what they need.

COMPASSIONATE REFLECTION

1. In your teaching, how do you support your students to have an individualized practice?
2. In your next class, what is one way that you could further encourage an individualized practice, or refine what you are already doing?

MOVING RHYTHMICALLY

While we have explored the benefits of encouraging our students to listen to their own needs and move and breathe in a way that reflects that, moving or practising together as a group can also be beneficial.

People often report feeling lonely when they are experiencing depression and anxiety,[1] and those who have experienced trauma often feel disconnected and out of sync with others.[2]

In his widely read book *The Body Keeps the Score*, Bessel van der Kolk writes about the importance of communal rhythms and synchronicity in healing from trauma,[3] and in *Overcoming Trauma through Yoga*, van der Kolk's colleagues Emerson and Hopper suggest creating intrapersonal and interpersonal rhythms in yoga classes to overcome this sense of disconnection and dyssynchrony with the self and other.[4] I have found that cueing for both interpersonal and intrapersonal rhythms can be a wonderful way to teach a class, cultivate a sense of community, tune into our own needs and practise moving back and forth between the needs or rhythms of the group and the needs and rhythms of the individual.

Let us take a look at *intra*personal and *inter*personal rhythms now.

Intrapersonal rhythms

In the context of a yoga class, an *intra*personal rhythm is a rhythm that we create internally, matching our movement to the breath. This can be a powerful way to self-regulate by tuning into our own internal rhythms and needs and moving in a way that is supportive of this.

When I began teaching yoga, I would often ask students to link their movements to the rhythm of their own breath, but that was all the instruction I gave them. On reflection, I do not think many of my students actually understood what this meant, and my other cues were more consistent with them linking their physical movements to the rhythm of *my* breath than of their own.

In a group class, it can be very easy to fall into the habit of telling students when to inhale and exhale. For example, in a standing forward fold we might instruct students to inhale with us and lift their hands above their head and then exhale together and fold forward.

Instead, we can encourage an intrapersonal rhythm by inviting our students to move with the rhythm of their own breath. With a standing forward fold, we could invite them to stand in a comfortable position with their arms by their sides, then wait until their inhalation arrives. And when it does, lift their arms overhead, filling the full length of the inhalation with the movement. Then wait for the exhalation and, when it arrives, fold forward, filling the full length of the exhalation with the forward folding movement.

If it is a more complex sequence, or a sequence that the class has not tried before, you might guide your students through the practice initially as a group, being more directive with cueing the breath (in an interpersonal rhythm). Then, once they have understood the sequence, invite them to practice in synchronization with their own breathing pattern (an intrapersonal rhythm).

Interpersonal rhythms

An *inter*personal rhythm is a rhythm that we create with others, matching our movements, breath or sounds. This can be a powerful way to foster a sense of connection and community. If you have ever been part of a choreographed group dance, chanted at a kirtan event or a football match or sung in a choir, you might know how powerful it can be to move, chant or sing together in synchronization with others.

When guiding a class to move or breathe together, be mindful of the pace and rhythm in the class, ensuring that it is slow enough so your students can follow along and be present in their bodies without feeling rushed, but not too slow, which could allow for drifting off or rumination.

Personally, I like to initially teach with an interpersonal rhythm, using both verbal and visual cues to introduce a new posture or sequence. This can help students to understand what I am teaching and gives them the experience of practising with others in the class. And when I sense that the students understand what I am offering and have had an experience of practising together, then I often switch to an intrapersonal rhythm, inviting students to practise in the rhythm of their own breath pattern, allowing them to tune inwards and find a way of practicing that is uniquely theirs. Students then get the experience of moving back and forth between being in community and tuning into their own internal needs, which is a powerful thing to practise, not only in the yoga room but in our communities.

COMPASSIONATE REFLECTION

1. Do you tend to teach more in a way that encourages interpersonal or intrapersonal rhythms?
2. What is one way that you could refine your teaching to include and encourage both interpersonal and intrapersonal rhythms?
3. Try it out, and then spend some time reflecting on how it went, including what went well, what did not go so well and how you would do it differently next time.

LANGUAGE

Using skilful and compassionate language can be a powerful therapeutic tool.

The language and tone we use when teaching and speaking to our students can be welcoming, uplifting and connecting, or it can be harmful, disconnecting and increase feelings of shame and body dissatisfaction.

Individuals experiencing depression and anxiety may hold core beliefs of not being good enough or likeable, and therefore may be hypervigilant to cues that confirm this bias. If we are not careful, our students may have these biases unconsciously confirmed in our yoga classes, and leave feeling worse than when they arrived.

Survivors of trauma may feel unsafe in the world, and are unlikely to feel comfortable or relaxed in your class unless they feel safe in your presence. They need to know that they can trust you.

To foster safety, welcoming and inclusion, a skilful yoga teacher can intentionally use language that is invitational, inclusive, non-judgemental, accurate, fosters connection and encourages curiosity and can avoid, or be mindful of, potentially triggering words. Let us explore these qualities now.

Invitational

Inviting your students to try a posture or a practice rather than *telling* them to do it or asking them to do it for *you*, can encourage self-empowerment and agency: a belief in one's ability to take effective action in the world.

Many people who have experienced trauma have had an experience of being forced to do something that they did not wish to do. And often when we are feeling depressed or anxious we also feel disempowered in our lives. So by inviting your students to make choices about their own yoga practice, they have the opportunity to have a lived experience of having agency and power over their own bodies and their own practice. And while this may sound like a small thing, it can be huge.

Instead of telling your students what to do, for example, 'move into Downward Facing Dog now', consider saying 'the invitation is to join me for Downward Facing Dog' or 'if it feels right for you, move into Downward Facing Dog' or 'if you like, you might choose to experiment with Downward Facing Dog'. There are so many different ways to share yoga using invitational language, the invitation is to experiment and play with it and find a way that feels right for you (see what I did there?!).

I have also heard many yoga teachers ask their students to do a posture or practice for *them*. Ideally, however, we want to support our students to practise for themselves, not for us, so consider avoiding language that asks students to do something on your behalf. Instead of saying, 'lift your leg for me', consider saying, 'if it feels right, the invitation is to lift your leg' or perhaps 'you might try lifting your leg, or alternatively leave it resting where it is, whatever feels best in your body in this moment. There is no right or wrong way of doing it.'

While using invitational rather than directive language can feel a little cumbersome to begin with, my experience has been that it gets easier and more natural with practice, and that students really warm to it. Students have told me they feel more empowered in the class and feel more accepted for themselves just as they are when their teachers have used invitational language.

Inclusive and non-judgemental

Using inclusive and non-judgemental language can be a powerful way to help our students to feel safe and welcome. Here are a few ways to make your language more inclusive and less judgemental when teaching.

Instead of telling your students about the *proper*, *advanced* or *full expression* of a practice and telling them they can do an *easier* version if they are unable to do the *full* version, try letting your students know that there are *different* variations of the practice, and encourage them to choose the variation that feels the most nourishing or most in alignment with their intention. This helps to communicate that all variations of the postures are equal (the objectively more *difficult* postures are not intrinsically *better*) and the variation they choose does not reflect their value or worth, or even how well they are doing the practice.

If a student is practising in a way that is different from the way you suggested, instead of calling out across the room to correct them, try letting it go and saying nothing at all; they might be doing the perfect practice for them in that moment. Or, if it looks unsafe or if they are looking to you for further direction, try discreetly offering them guidance about how to make the practice more stable or more to their needs. As we explored in the section on touch, the more we let go of the idea that postures or practices need to look a certain way, or that there is a *right* or *wrong* way of doing yoga, the less need there is for corrections at all.

Using language that is body positive can communicate that everyone and everybody is welcome. Instead of offering postures or sequences to *get in shape*, to *get a six-pack* or to *lose weight*, consider avoiding talking about the body in a way that values a particular body-type or objectifies the body at all. If you notice yourself speaking to yourself or others in a way that objectifies the body, it could be an indication that you might need to explore your own relationship with your body. In the world we live in, it is pretty difficult not to have a dysfunctional relationship with our bodies, so it's important that we do our own work around this and are mindful not to perpetuate this dysfunction in our yoga classes.

Consider avoiding referring to a practice as *easy*, as what might be easy for you could be very difficult for someone else, and it can be very demoralizing to hear something that you are struggling with called *easy*. Instead, try offering different variations of a practice, or encouraging students to find a way of practising that works for them.

Instead of presuming someone's gender by their name or by way they look, consider using gender-neutral language (for example, 'welcome everyone' rather than 'welcome ladies'). Consider also adding a field for pronouns on your intake form and introducing yourself at the beginning of class and online using your pronouns to create a culture of inclusivity and respect for people's gender identities.

I have only touched on a few of the ways that we can use language to make our classes more inclusive and non-judgemental; this could be an entire book on its own. We go into more detail in the Mental Health Aware Yoga training.

Curiosity

Consider inviting your students to be curious about what they are experiencing, rather than telling them what to do or how to feel in a particular practice.

For example, instead of telling your students what to do by saying, 'raise your arms', you could you invite them to be curious about the experience of raising their arms. For example, you could say, 'notice what happens when you raise your arms' or 'feel what arises within you when you raise your arms' or 'experiment with raising your arms' or 'what would it feel like if you raised your arms here?'

Annabel McLisky, a yoga teacher of 45 years, retired psychologist, co-founder of Trauma Sensitive Yoga Australia and Mental Health Aware Yoga Mentor, told me recently that the word *notice* is one of the most useful words she draws on when teaching yoga. She will often say: 'Notice how this feels in your body, noticing without judgement or criticism. Your body is clever, it will let you know how it feels. Feel free to adjust your position according to what you are feeling in your body, always moving away from discomfort and towards comfort.'

In addition, when we tell a student how they *should* feel in a practice, especially if it is a very positive experience, students can feel like they are doing the practice incorrectly or are having the wrong response to the practice if they feel differently. For example, hearing a teacher say, 'feel awakened and alive' or 'feel gratitude for your life', when they are feeling exhausted and depressed and are working out how to leave an emotionally abusive relationship may result in your student feeling like *they* are wrong in some way, and they may beat themselves up or disconnect from you and the class.

So, instead of saying, for example, 'you should feel strong and powerful in this posture' or 'feel your heart opening to love', consider saying, 'if it's helpful, notice what you feel in this posture' or (one of my favourites) 'perhaps notice the effects of this practice on your body, breath and mind'.

This can gently encourage self-enquiry (getting to know yourself just as you are) and distress tolerance (the ability to tolerate uncomfortable emotional and physical states).

However, not everyone will be able to sense their internal sensations, particularly if they have experienced significant trauma. So consider using invitational language when inviting students to notice, being more specific about where they may notice sensation (for example, 'noticing how this feels in the shoulder') and letting them know that it's okay not to notice anything. I like to say 'perhaps noticing sensation, or the absence of sensation' to include the possibility of students experiencing sensation or nothing at all.

Many of us, especially during challenging times, find it difficult to tolerate our internal experience and may try to deny, suppress or get rid of our unwanted sensations, emotions and thoughts. Gently inviting students to be curious about their unfolding internal experiences can support them to notice them, rather than suppress or attempt to change them, which can be an important part in cultivating positive mental health.

We do need to be careful about encouraging students experiencing heightened states of arousal to stay with an emotion or sensation that they are experiencing, and this is best done one-on-one with an experienced therapist. However, as yoga teachers, we can plant the seeds for this by inviting our students to be curious of their internal experience, particularly the body (annamaya kosha) and the breath (prāṇāmaya kosha).

Connection

Connection is a powerful human experience and can be incredibly life-affirming and healing. In your yoga classes, try using language that supports students to foster a connection with themselves, with you, with others in the class and, if it is appropriate, with God or something higher than ourselves.

To help your students to connect with themselves you might encourage an individualized practice and intrapersonal rhythms, as we explored earlier in this chapter. Instead of telling them to push through and keep going, even when they are tired or in pain, try inviting your students to connect inwardly with themselves, to listen to their bodies and practise in a way that is most in alignment with their needs in each moment and with their intention for their practice.

To support the connection with you, the teacher, try authentically greeting students when they arrive, asking and being available for them to check in with you before and after class, using people's names when you can and being supportive of all students, no matter how flexible, strong or experienced they are. Connection is also naturally fostered when we use language that is invitational, non-judgemental, curious and inclusive.

Instead of using the standard greeting of 'hi, how are you?' without pausing for the answer (as we do so often in English speaking countries), consider only asking this question if you are prepared to do so with sincerity and can take the time to listen to a real answer. A question that is more likely to elicit a genuine response, especially in the short amount of time we often have before a class and with other people around, is, 'what would you like to get out of, or focus on, in class today?' Their answer can also help to inform the direction of your class.

Using your students' names and greeting them individually can be a simple but often very connecting experience. Do not underestimate the power of this!

Accurate

As best you can, be accurate and precise with your language and avoid commenting on areas outside your area of expertise.

It can be confusing to hear a teacher say, 'breathe into your big toe' when this is clearly impossible. The student may either spend the class trying to work out how to breathe into their big toe and feel dismayed when they are unable to do it, or dismiss you as not knowing what you are talking about. This does not mean that you cannot use analogies or metaphors; the goal is to be clear in your language. Instead, try saying something like, 'imagine your breath extending down into your big toe'.

Avoid triggering words

Certain words and phrases have the potential to be triggering for some students, particularly those who have experienced trauma.

The reality is that any word has the potential to be triggering, and it is just not possible to completely eradicate triggering words from our vocabulary. We are all different, with different cultural, familial, individual and trauma experiences. Something that feels supportive and encouraging to you, could feel triggering and unsafe to me, and vice versa.

As a result, it is important that we use our words mindfully, avoiding the use of potentially triggering words as best we can and that we continually listen and learn from our students about what works and what does not work for them.

Here are some examples of words or phrases that may be triggering:

- bend over
- hang your head
- hang in there
- once you have the hang of it
- stroke your inner thigh
- place your hands on your booty
- sit your butt down
- lift your nipples to the sky
- muscles melting away from the bone
- touch yourself
- root yourself into the ground (in Australia *root* also means rough sex)
- I will come around now and tuck you in (e.g. with a blanket in Śavāsana or Corpse Pose)
- good girl/boy
- Sexy Cat (for modified Marjaryāsana-Bitilāsana or Cat/Cow Pose)
- Hello Honey Pose (for Ananda Balāsana or Happy Baby Pose)
- imagine your mother supporting you
- Corpse Pose
- Easy Pose
- pose.

While I hope it is clear why most of the phrases on this list have the potential to be triggering, what might not be obvious is the final word, *pose.*

This word may have negative connotations for someone who has experienced sexual or physical abuse, may communicate that yoga postures are about *posing* or displaying oneself in a certain way and that there is a right or wrong way of doing the yoga practices. Therefore, consider avoiding using the word *pose*, especially when you know there are students in your class who have experienced abuse. Instead, you could use words like *posture, practice, form* or *shape.*

There is a lot of information covered in this section on language. If you are new to teaching, I know that it can feel overwhelming to try to get it *right* and not say the *wrong* thing, and, if you have been teaching for a long time, it can be difficult to undo some of the teaching phrases that roll off the tongue automatically. But I also know that we can change habits and obtain skills through repetition and practice. If you would like to, try choosing one phrase that you would like to bring into your teaching, and then thread it into your language as you teach. Keep doing it until you have found a way that works for you and feels second nature; then add another one, and so on. Over time, you will develop a mental health aware lexicon that feels and sounds natural and is nourishing and supportive for your students.

In conclusion, while I do encourage you to be conscious of your language and skilful in the way that you use it, you do not need to be anxious and hypervigilant about saying the *wrong* thing. If we create a safe container for our students, then a student may feel safe enough to tolerate and even gain insight from words or phrases that they experience as triggering during class.

COMPASSIONATE REFLECTION

1. Which of these words or phrases are triggering for you?
2. Which of these words or phrases have the potential to be triggering for your students?

3. What other words or phrases would you add to the list of triggering words?
4. Is there a word or phrase that you read in this section that you would like to remove or bring into your teaching? Try it out, then reflect on how it felt for you to use this language and for your students to hear.

EMBODIMENT

Many of us *live in our heads* or in the case of dissociation, feel like we are living outside or above our heads. As a result of the high value placed on the intellect in many educational and work domains, many of us were taught from childhood to ignore or override the messages and signals that our bodies give us. It is no wonder that so many of us feel disembodied.

Embodiment refers to being present to the unfolding sensations and messages of the body, and helps us to be more in the present moment.

Clinical psychologist and yoga teacher Bo Forbes describes embodiment as a continuum from exteroception to proprioception to interoception.[5]

Exteroception is the awareness of what is happening in the world around us, using our senses to gather this information.[6]

Proprioception is the awareness of the body in space, knowing where other people and objects are and the relative size and movement of our own body.[7] Yoga teachers will often give proprioceptive cues in class, and experienced yoga practitioners will often have a well-developed sense of proprioception.

Interoception is the awareness of our internal state, and is the process of receiving, accessing and appraising internal bodily signals[8].

Cueing all three, exteroception, proprioception and interoception, can be helpful at different times in a yoga class.

Cueing exteroception (for example, noticing what objects are present in the room), may help someone to feel grounded and safe in their surrounds. In the 5,4,3,2,1 Grounding Practice you will read about in the Mental Health Crisis chapter, the first part of the practice is a cue to facilitate exteroception, with the invitation to notice five things you can see in the room.

Cueing proprioception (for example noticing where the feet are placed and where the arms are located in space), may help someone to be aware of where their body is located, help to ensure their alignment is safe and support them to move from a dissociated state back into their body.

And cueing interoception (for example noticing the way a practice feels in the body), can support someone to be aware of and to tolerate their internal experience, and to take action based on their internal cues.

Benefits of embodiment

Embodiment can help us to live more in the present moment. The mind has a tendency to ruminate and wander into the past or future, and by noticing or sensing the physical sensations of the body, we can anchor ourselves more steadily in the present moment.

In addition, by tuning into our internal experience, we can gain insight into our needs and wants and, in turn, take aligned action based on these. Often, individuals with depression, anxiety or a history of trauma feel like they have very little agency in the world, so supporting them to come home to their bodies can support them to rediscover this.

Fostering embodiment through yoga

In the yoga class we can gently and subtly support our students to attend, trust and come home to their bodies as we focus not just on exteroception and proprioception but also, if it feels okay, on non-judgemental and compassionate interoception.

As Bessel van der Kolk says, '[y]oga turns out to be a terrific way to (re)gain a relationship with the interior world and with it a caring, loving, sensual relationship to the self.'[9]

There are many ways that we can foster interoceptive embodiment when teaching yoga, including slowing the class down to allow students the opportunity to sense their internal experience, inviting a quality of gentle curiosity rather than expecting things to be a certain way and inviting our students to notice or sense their internal experience while practising. For example, you could invite students to try 'sensing the movement of the breath in the body' or 'noticing the effect this practice has on your feet'.

While noticing and sensing emotions (manomaya kosha) and thoughts (vijnānamaya kosha) can be a powerful practice, staying within the first two koshas, the body (annamaya kosha) and breath (prāṇāmaya kosha), is likely to feel safer and more accessible for students experiencing mental health challenges, and is more within the scope of practice of a yoga teacher when teaching students who are experiencing mental health challenges (unless they also have dual qualifications as a mental health professional).

While invitations for interoception and embodiment can be a powerful way to support recovery from mental illness, it also has the potential to be confusing, difficult or overwhelming for some, particularly if challenging sensations, emotions or thoughts arise. If it is appropriate for the students you are teaching, consider offering invitations for interoception and embodiment, with the focus on the body and the breath, and always with the option of disregarding your invitations if they do not make sense or feel okay.

COMPASSIONATE REFLECTION

1. Look around you now. What can you notice in your environment (exteroception)?
2. How is your body positioned now? Where are your arms and legs in space (proprioception)?
3. What internal sensations can you feel (interoception)?
4. When you are teaching yoga, do you generally use exteroceptive, proprioceptive or interoceptive cues?

5. After reading this section on embodiment, is there anything that you would like to try out in your teaching?
6. Try it, then spend some time reflecting on how it went, including what went well, what did not go so well and what you would do differently next time.

Pillar Five

YOGIC PRACTICES

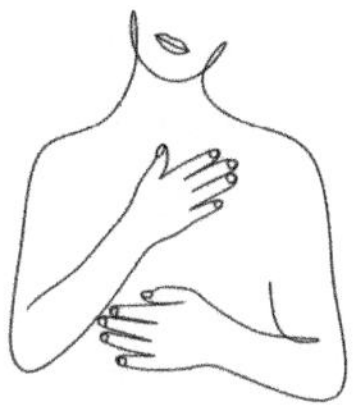

Yoga provides an exquisite toolkit for regulating our nervous system, managing our mental health and cultivating sattva.

There is a vast array of yoga practices that can be immensely helpful in supporting us to down-regulate (calm) when we are feeling anxious, hyper-aroused or rajasic, to up-regulate (activate) when we are feeling depressed, hypo-aroused or tamasic and to return to, or stay within, what Siegel termed the Window of Tolerance, or sattva.

In this chapter, we will explore āsana, prāṇāyāma and meditation practices for cultivating sattva.

YOGA AND MENTAL HEALTH RESEARCH

While there have been many studies in the past few decades examining the effects of yoga on mental health, the challenge with researching yoga is that it is either too broad to define and therefore difficult to research using our current scientific methodology, or that it has been reduced down to a single practice or protocol which could be considered reductionistic, representing only a limited part of the entirety of yoga.

And when yoga is reduced down to a particular protocol or set of practices to fit the current scientific method, the research shows a wide variety of yoga practices, without consensus of what actually constitutes yoga. Some studies include only āsana, others only prāṇāyāma, or only meditation, mantra, mudra or kriyā, and others include a combination of all of these and more.

While there have been some high-quality randomized clinical trials (the gold standard in research) investigating yoga and mental health, there are various methodological limitations in the research, including small sample sizes, uncontrolled designs (e.g. single group trials) and heterogeneity of controls and interventions, and therefore more good quality, evidence-based research is still required.[1,2]

Despite all this, overall, the contemporary evidence suggests that yoga, either in a group or one-on-one, can help with mental health, particularly as an adjunct to treatment.[3]

We also need to remember that yoga has been practised and researched for thousands of years. It was an evidence-based practice long before the contemporary scientific method arose. Unlike many contemporary psychological treatments which have only been around for a few years or decades, yoga has been around for many years, and has been trialled by goodness knows how many people during this time, many of whom I imagine had a much greater understanding of the human condition than most contemporary researchers working under stressful conditions in universities!

Just because the ancient yogis did not use SPSS (the statistical analysis software used by many researchers today) for the analysis of their data, it does not mean that yoga has not been rigorously tested and examined for its efficacy.

I am not saying that we should ignore the contemporary scientific method, not at all. If you take the Mental Health Aware Yoga training, you will learn about some of the key research from the last decade. However, I do think that we need to be aware of colonized scientific practices, and to be careful not to dismiss the thousands of years of practice and research that has gone into yogic methods just because they were not published in a contemporary scientific journal.

ASSESSING YOUR STUDENTS

In order to share yoga practices and sequence our classes intelligently, we first need to understand our students' current mental health state.

Some students will be very open and simply tell you about their mental health. I am noticing more and more how open many people are becoming about their mental health and their struggles. Some students will tell you about a recent diagnosis by their mental health professional or let you know that they are feeling a bit down or a bit anxious at the start of class.

Even if they do not explicitly tell you, you can get a sense of your students' mental health state through the lens of the guṇas, and this can inform *how* and *what* you teach. Remember the guṇas? We explored rajas, tamas and sattva and their correlation to mental health in the Yoga Psychology chapter.

When teaching, try noticing the way your students arrive at your class, the speed they speak and move at, their posture, breath and the way they hold their bodies.

When you check in with your students individually as they arrive, listen to what they tell you about how they are feeling. They may not use the words rajas, tamas or sattva, but they might say that they are feeling a bit tired or flat (tamas) or feeling worked up about something (rajas) or feeling calm (sattva).

Notice if students are striving for perfection during class (rajas), if they are giving up easily (tamas) or if they are practising in a way that matches their intention and ability (sattva). Or perhaps if they show a preference for a strong dynamic practice (rajas), a gentle restorative practice (tamas) or a balanced practice that suits their individual needs (sattva).

All of these factors can help to inform you which of the guṇas may be predominant and will assist you in selecting the most appropriate practices, or variations of practices, for your students.

Whether you are teaching a group or an individual session, starting your class in a similar way each time can be a great way to help you to read the room and understand your students' needs, as you use this as a baseline and learn to gauge your students' mental health based on how students respond.

From a mental health perspective, here is an overview of how the guṇas may present in your students in a yoga class:

RAJAS	TAMAS	SATTVA
Anxious or angry energy	Depressive energy	Content and calm energy
Hyper-aroused	Hypo-aroused	Within the Window of Tolerance or optimum zone of arousal[4]
Agitated, stressed or busy	Exhausted, overwhelmed, sad or shut down	Calm and happy
Arriving early or arriving late and rushing into class	Arriving late and moving slowly into class, with obvious effort	Arriving mindfully and at the appropriate time
Speaking quickly	Speaking slowly	Speaking calmly
Moving quickly	Moving slowly	Moving calmly
Moving continuously	Moving as little as possible	Moving as required
Tense and restless body posture	Stooped shoulders and collapsed chest	Calm posture
Tension in the face, including the jaw, brow and around the eyes	Expressionless face	Calm face
Looking around the room	Looking down	Looking inwards and at the teacher
Breath fast and shallow, chest breathing, holding the breath	Breath shallow or looking like they are barely breathing, sighing	Breath easy and rhythmic, diaphragmatic breathing
Preferring a strong dynamic practice	Preferring a slow, gentle restorative practice	Preferring a balanced practice that suits their individual needs
Perfectionistic, striving to get practices *right*	Disinterest, giving up easily	Practising in alignment with their intention and ability
Feeling frustrated if they do not get postures *right*	Feeling disheartened and hopeless if they do not get postures *right*	Content with their ability in each posture, there is no *right*
Easily irritated or angry	Cry easily	Calm

Anticipating the next practice before the teacher gives an instruction	Losing track of the teacher's instructions, daydreaming	Listening attentively to the teacher's instructions
Choosing what they perceive is the most advanced variation of the practice	Choosing the variation of the practice that requires the least effort	Choosing the variation of the practice that suits their individual needs in each moment
Asking lots of questions	Not asking any questions	Asking questions occasionally when relevant
Difficulty sleeping (unable to get to sleep, night-waking or waking too early in the morning)	Over-sleeping (difficulty getting out of bed in the morning)	Restorative sleep (wakes feeling refreshed)
Restless in Śavāsana	Falling asleep in Śavāsana	At ease in Śavāsana

To be clear, it is not the role of the yoga teacher to diagnosis mental illness, and you cannot know definitively which guṇa is predominant for your students; however, you can take a pretty good guess about the guṇas by carefully noticing your students and listening to what they tell you, then use this hypothesis, not to diagnose your students, but to design the class.

Ideally, we would also support our students to tune into their own needs, and come to their own conclusions about their internal state and what they need from their practice.

COMPASSIONATE REFLECTION

1. Which guṇas are typically predominant in your students?
2. Do your classes tend to attract predominantly one of the guṇas, or is there a variety of presentations?
3. Which of the examples provided do you see most?

SHARING YOGA PRACTICES

We can support our students to maintain their mental health, overcome mental health challenges and cultivate sattva by teaching yoga in a way that is intentionally designed to increase sattva, reduce tamas and rajas, and is mindful of contraindications for depression, anxiety, stress and trauma.

We can do this in the following ways:

- Share specific practices to increase sattva and reduce tamas and rajas in class, including āsana, prāṇāyāma and meditation.
- Offer variations of practices that focus more on reducing tamas or reducing rajas (this can be particularly helpful in a group setting) where you teach one practice to the whole class and offer different variations, depending on the students' needs.
- Share information about potential benefits of the practices we teach, and encourage students to practice outside the yoga class.
- Avoid, or provide psychoeducation about practices that have the potential to be triggering or imbalancing for students experiencing mental health challenges.

In addition to feeling the benefits in class, giving our students the yogic tools to self-regulate and information about when and how to utilize them can be incredibly empowering. This can result in an increased sense of self-efficacy, as our students learn to rely on themselves to effect change in their lives, rather than relying on their yoga teacher or therapist.

It is important, however, that we only discuss *possible* or *potential* benefits, always inviting students to try the practices out and experience the effects themselves. We do not ever want to presume that a practice will have a particular effect on our students. We are all different, and we can never really know the effect a practice will have on an individual student. We can communicate what the effect might be based on our own experience or on research, but always with the disclaimer that we are all different and we need to find the practices that work for us.

In the following sections you will find specific practices that can assist in increasing the predominance of sattva and reducing the predominance of tamas and rajas.

And because knowing what *not* to teach is arguably just as important as knowing what to teach, you will also find some important contraindications and precautions for individuals experiencing depression, anxiety, stress and trauma. As a rule of thumb, the more severe a students' mental health challenges are, the more important it will be to avoid the contraindicated practices and cues and go very gently when sharing any yoga practices.

This is not an exhaustive list of practices and contraindications but rather a great starting point. We go into much more detail in the Mental Health Aware Yoga training.

Before sharing any of these practices with students, the invitation is to try them out on yourself and notice the effects they have on your body, breath and mind. And if you do share them with your students, invite them to notice the effects of the practices, and to experiment with them in class and in their home practice to really make them their own.

PRACTICES FOR CULTIVATING SATTVA

Yoga has an abundance of practices and sequences that can help us to up-regulate or energize when we are feeling tamasic or hypo-aroused, and practices to down-regulate or calm when we are feeling rajasic or hyper-aroused.

We will explore these up- and down-regulating practices later in this chapter; however, there are many yoga practices and sequences that can help us to cultivate sattva and reduce *both* tamas and rajas (how magic is that?!). It is here where we will begin.

Āsana

Contrary to what many people believe, the focus when practising āsana for mental health is less on *what* you practise, and more about *how* you practise it. In this section, we will explore some ideas on *how* to share āsana with your students to support the cultivation of sattva, as well as a couple of specific āsanas that may be helpful.

In whatever āsana or sequence of āsanas you are sharing, try

co-ordinating the movement with the breath, rather than the other way around, as we explored in the Therapeutic Skills chapter. This can be an incredible way to regulate the nervous system and cultivate more sattva.

For a simple, accessible and embodied way to introduce this concept, try inviting your students to sit or stand, in any comfortable position, then inhale and lift the arms overhead, then exhale to bring the arms back by their sides. Guide your students through this a few times together, creating an *interpersonal* rhythm with the whole class (or with you if you are teaching a private session).

Once your students are comfortable with this, try inviting them to leave their arms by their sides and wait for the inhalation to arrive, and, only when it naturally arises inviting them to lift their arms, filling the full length of the breath with the movement. And with the arms overhead, inviting them to wait for the exhalation, and when it arrives, to lower the arms by their sides, again filling the full length of the exhalation with the movement. You could invite your students to repeat this three (or more) times, linking the movement of the arms with the rhythm of their own breath, thus creating an *intrapersonal* rhythm.

Watch me teaching this sequence at www.mentalhealthawareyoga.com/book-resources.

Consider also letting your students know in advance **how many times** you will be inviting them to repeat the practice, and that they are welcome to practise for a longer or shorter amount of time as they choose. This reinforces choice, helps the sequence to be predictable, lets students know when it will end and gives students autonomy over their own practice.

Cueing for interoception and embodiment is another way that can be helpful in cultivating sattva, as we explored in the Therapeutic Skills chapter. If it is appropriate for your students, consider using language that emphasizes inhabiting the body and sensing or being curious about what is unfolding internally during movement and while holding āsanas. Instead of telling people what to feel, either physically, emotionally or energetically, try inviting them to sense or notice what is unfolding (sensation or the absence of sensation) instead.

You can do this in any āsana or sequence you teach; however, sensing or noticing is often more accessible when teaching a slower pace.

Two types of āsanas that may be beneficial in cultivating sattva when either rajas *or* tamas is dominant are Vīrabhadrāsanas (Warrior Poses) and balancing postures such as Vṛkṣāsana (Tree Pose).

Vīrabhadrāsanas may help to embody strength and grounding. I have found in my own practice that I naturally begin to feel stronger and more grounded when I practise one of the Vīrabhadrāsana variations, even if I am not thinking about the rationale behind them or trying to consciously embody these qualities. Simply offering these warrior postures may support students to feel strong and grounded. There may be no need to name the potential benefits at all, and, indeed, by not naming them, you will be less likely to ostracize anyone who might not be feeling these qualities when they practise. Instead you might invite people to *notice* how they feel when practising one of these āsanas.

In a similar way, balancing postures, such as Vṛkṣāsana, may help students to feel strong and to stabilize the mind. Have you ever noticed how difficult it can be to think and balance at the same time? Try it out for yourself and notice what happens!

Balancing postures can be great way to help a busy and ruminative mind to cut through the mind-chatter and develop one-pointed focus, even if just for a second or two. Attending to proprioception (awareness of the position of the body in space) and interoception (the unfolding sensations within the body) requires even more focus, and it may therefore be even more difficult to think about other things while practising. So, if it is appropriate for your students, consider both proprioceptive and interoceptive cues when sharing a balancing practice. However, be sure not to overwhelm them with too many cues!

Vṛkṣāsana can also be a great time to share a little psychoeducation about balancing and the mind. As students finish the practice on one leg, try giving them information about balancing and the mind during the transition to the other leg and invite them to be curious about their own experience of balancing and thinking as they practice on the other leg. It is important to be aware that everyone will have a different experience of this, and some people *will* be able to balance and ruminate at the same time. Always share this information, and any other information about practices, in a way that invites people to try it out and gather evidence for themselves as to what is helpful or unhelpful for them.

Contraindications and precautions for āsana

Students with a history of trauma may be triggered by **intense physical āsanas**, so if you are working with survivors of trauma, consider offering more gentle postures.

In his first research study with yoga for trauma survivors, medical doctor and author of *The Body Keeps the Score*, Bessel van der Kolk, and colleagues had a drop-out rate of 50%, the highest drop-out rate they had ever experienced in their research. When they interviewed the participants who had dropped out of the classes, they learned that the yoga program was too intense and that postures that involved the pelvis could precipitate intense panic or flashbacks of sexual assault. In subsequent research, they slowed the yoga practice down to 'a snail's pace' and, following the change, only one of the 35 participants dropped out.[5]

Van der Kolk hypothesized that 'intense physical sensations unleashed the demons from the past that had been so carefully kept in check by numbing and inattention'[6], and so they were careful to share more gentle yoga practices in the future.

If you are teaching people who you know have had an experience of trauma, learn from the mistakes of van der Kolk and colleagues and consider teaching a gentle and slow class.

This does not mean that you should never offer strong practices in your classes, but if you know (or suspect) that the students you are teaching have a history of trauma, it would likely be wise to offer more gentle postures and practices instead. If you do offer strong postures in a general class, be mindful of always offering alternatives and be aware of the potential for stronger or more dynamic postures to be triggering for some students, as a strong posture was for me in a yoga class after the Bourke Street incident I shared in the Western Psychology chapter.

While **cueing for interoception** and inviting students to notice sensation in the body can be helpful for some, for those who are experiencing moderate to severe mental illness or those who cannot tolerate their emotions and associated sensations, it has the potential to be overwhelming or triggering. So, unless you are a mental health professional who feels confident working in these domains, keep the focus on the body (annamaya kosha) and the breath (prāṇāmaya kosha), rather than on emotions (manomaya kosha) and thoughts (vijnānamaya kosha). Be sure to also let students know that sensing the body is always optional and they can ignore these invitations if they are not helpful for them. If you notice that your students are being triggered or overwhelmed by cues to sense the body, adapt your teaching and consider leaving these cues out. As I mentioned previously, I like to invite students to 'notice sensation or the absence of sensation' to help make these interoceptive cues more inclusive, so students do not feel like they are doing something wrong if they cannot feel or sense anything. In addition, as some students can become confused by open invitations to sense the body, it can be helpful to give students more directive interoceptive cues, inviting them to notice sensation in a particular part of the body, where sensation is most likely to be felt (for example, in the feet in a standing position, or in the shoulders when the arms are lifted).

If we are not careful, guiding an āsana class can **sound regimented and controlling**. If we tell students precisely when and how to move and breathe, this may be triggering for individuals who have an experience of trauma that involved being controlled. It can also encourage students to override their own instincts about their body, which is the opposite of what we want to do. Instead, consider teaching in a way that is invitational, inclusive, non-judgemental, accurate, fosters connection and encourages curiosity (as we explored in the language section) and be mindful of everything in the Safe Container and Therapeutic Skills chapters.

When teaching a class with trauma survivors, consider **avoiding using yoga straps** and avoiding teaching in studios that have ropes or yoga straps hanging from the wall, like you see in some Iyengar Yoga studios. For someone who has experienced trauma that involved being tied up or restrained, or has attempted suicide through hanging or knows someone who has, this could be very confronting and overwhelming.

However, yoga straps can make some āsanas more accessible for students, so I do not believe that we need to avoid the use of straps entirely, particularly if we are teaching in a more generalized setting. However, even if you are teaching in a setting where no one has disclosed a history of trauma, statistically it is likely that at least one of your students has experienced trauma, so it is important to be sensitive to this when introducing straps in your classes.

If you do choose to use yoga straps, I suggest always offering a variation that does not include the strap and inviting your students to consider using the strap on themselves, rather than you tying or wrapping them in it. Consider demonstrating on yourself first, so the students know what to expect, and letting them know how long the practice will last, so they know that it will come to an end. Students who are triggered by using straps or by seeing other students in the class use the straps may be able to tolerate it if they are in control of the strap themselves and they know exactly what is going to happen and when it will end.

If you are teaching Restorative Yoga or offering extra props in Śavāsana, try inviting students to **organize their own blankets** and bolsters, rather than you putting the blankets over them and tucking them in. This not only teaches your students how to do it themselves so they can continue to practise outside of the yoga class, but is also less likely to be triggering for a student who experienced abuse in bed where they may have been tucked in at night by a perpetrator.

Be aware that **Ananda Balāsana** (Happy Baby Pose) can be triggering for some people, especially if they have had an experience of sexual abuse. In their research on yoga for individuals with trauma, van der Kolk and Emerson found that while Ananda Balāsana was triggering for some students, it was helpful for others when they could overcome their fear and do the posture calmly. They concluded that it was only appropriate to teach the posture when taught very gently and while encouraging students not to try it if it made them feel uncomfortable.[7]

I personally do not teach this āsana, but I am surprised at the number of students who choose to practice Ananda Balāsana when I invite them to choose their own practice towards the end of the āsana part of the class. If you do teach Ananda Balāsana in a group class, consider configuring the mats in a circle at the beginning of class and inviting the students to lie with their heads in the middle of the circle for this practice. So, if they choose to join you for Ananda Balāsana, they will not have anyone in front or behind them and will only be *exposing* themselves to the wall behind them, which may be less triggering.[8]

Prāṇāyāma

Prāṇāyāma can be incredibly helpful for students experiencing mental illness, but it can also be challenging and triggering. Keeping it simple and staying attentive to the effects it is having on your students is key.

I believe that the most important part, and ideally the first stage of any prāṇāyāma practice, is to **notice and sense the breath** just as it is, without trying to change it in any way. As Bessel van der Kolk says, '[m] any of our patients are barely aware of their breath, so learning to focus on the in and out breath, to notice whether the breath was fast or slow, and to count the breaths in some poses can be a significant accomplishment.'[9] We are all so used to trying to change our internal experience, through food, drugs, alcohol or technology, or even through yoga, that many of us have forgotten how to be present with ourselves.

Sensing the breath, and therefore being present with ourselves, can be a new and profound experience for many people. Being present with ourselves, just as we are, is a truly radical act of presence and self-acceptance. How often do we allow ourselves to be and accept ourselves just as we are, without trying to fix, improve or change anything? Life can sometimes feel like a constant self-improvement project with no end in sight. Sometimes, simply sensing the breath, just as it is, is all the prāṇāyāma practice that we need; it acknowledges a willingness to be with ourselves, just as we are.

Two different ways to notice the breath include sensing and listening to the breath.

My favourite way to work with the breath is to simply notice and **sense the breath** in the body. This is my go-to when I am feeling stressed or overwhelmed. I am a big fan of simple.

Try inviting your students to notice or sense the movement of the breath in the body wherever it is most vivid for them: in the nostrils, back of the throat, the chest or in the abdomen. They could also place their hands on their abdomen, ribs or chest to assist with noticing. This could be a very short practice of 10 seconds or a much longer practice, depending on the needs and capacity of the student.

Listening to the breath can be another accessible way to begin practising prāṇāyāma. Students who are disconnected from their bodies through trauma or through an overly intellectual existence may find it difficult or intolerable to feel the movement of the breath in the body, so inviting them to listen to the breath can be a safer and more accessible way for them to experience it.

You might suggest to your students that they listen for the sound of the breath in the nostrils or the back of the throat; doing so can naturally create a gentle Ujjāyī Prāṇāyāma-type sound. Not everyone will be able to hear their breath, so be sure to always let your students know that it is okay if they cannot hear it. Remember, not all practices are for everyone, and we do not want students to think that they cannot do yoga if they cannot hear or sense their breath.

If the only breath practice you taught your students was listening to, noticing or sensing the breath, oftentimes that would be enough. It is a simple but powerful practice, so be sure not to underestimate it. However, while it may be relatively simple, it will not be easy for everyone.

If your students are comfortable with noticing and sensing the breath, you might decide to offer prāṇāyāma practices to *regulate* the breath. However, for many students, and especially those with significant mental health challenges, being aware of and getting acquainted with the rhythm of the breath may be all that they can tolerate and all that is needed.

To share **abdominal or diaphragmatic breathing** with your students, invite them to feel the movement of the breath in their abdomen; the abdomen rising or expanding with the inhalation and releasing or gently contracting with the exhalation.

For some students, placing their hands on their abdomen or ribs can be helpful in providing extra sensory feedback. It can sometimes be easier for the abdomen to move freely when lying down, so consider offering this prāṇāyāma practice in a lying down position or during Śavāsana.

Even though the research tells us diaphragmatic breathing is helpful in reducing stress and anxiety,[10] some people find it difficult or impossible. So, as with all yoga practices, be sure to only offer this as a suggestion, and invite students to cease practising if they feel uncomfortable or disturbed at any time.

Another way to begin to regulate the breath is a simple instruction to **regulate the breath to be calm and steady**.

Try it out for yourself; it is surprising how effective this simple cue can be. As it is a fairly open instruction, without confusing breathing patterns or mudras to use, it may be effective for students who are new to yoga, those who find yoga a bit strange, those who tend to get confused or flustered easily or those who have had their breath controlled during a traumatic experience. In this prāṇāyāma practice they are in full control of the timing and the experience of regulating the breath.

Sama Vṛitti Prāṇāyāma, or Equal Breathing, is a gentle prāṇāyāma practice to equalize the length of the inhalation and exhalation. A longer inhalation is thought to activate the sympathetic (fight or flight) branch[11] of the autonomic nervous system and an extended exhalation to activate the parasympathetic (rest and digest) branch.[12]

Sama Vṛitti Prāṇāyāma can provide a balance between sympathetic and parasympathetic effects and can be a great starting point for lengthening either the inhalation or exhalation, depending on the needs of the student (more on this in the sections on practices for reducing rajas and tamas).

There are many ways that you can guide your students to equalize the breath. One way is to simply invite your students to make their inhalations and exhalations the same length. Another is to invite your students to count four counts on the inhalation and four counts on the exhalation.

When equalizing the breath through counting, I find it helpful to start with an interpersonal rhythm, where I count four counts on the inhalation aloud to guide the pace of the practice and to a rhythm that I hope will work for most people (always with the invitation to only join in with my counting if it feels right for them), and then move to an intrapersonal rhythm, inviting students to count in the rhythm of their own breath.

Nāḍī Sodhana Prāṇāyāma, or Alternate Nostril Breathing, is another prāṇāyāma practice that can be both balancing and calming. From a yogic perspective, this practice is designed to balance the iḍā and piṅgalā nāḍīs, the channels through the body in which prāṇā can leave and enter. Iḍā nāḍī passes through the left nostril and represents the cool energy of the moon (candra), and piṅgalā nāḍī passes through the right nostril and represents the hot energy of the sun (sūrya).[13]

This description lines up with contemporary autonomic nervous system research, which has found that left nostril breathing is associated with parasympathetic (calming) activity, and right nostril breathing with sympathetic (activating) activity.[14] Research has found that alternate nostril breathing has a complex but balancing effect on these systems,[15] with a tilt towards parasympathetic dominance.[16]

I suggest only teaching Nāḍī Sodhana Prāṇāyāma to students who have previous experience with breathing practices and are comfortable with sensing and regulating the breath. Start slowly, with perhaps one or two rounds, and build it up over time in accordance with the students' ability and preference.

Bhrāmarī Prāṇāyāma, or Humming Bee Breath, is a balancing practice that can be both calming and energizing. While there is limited research on its effectiveness for mental health, Bhrāmarī Prāṇāyāma has been found to promote parasympathetic activation[17,18,19] (possibly due to the extended exhalation) with mild uplifting effects on different physiological systems.[20] In addition, the sound, especially when the fingers are gently pressed into the outer cartilage of the ear, can help to create a focus for the mind, potentially cutting through ruminative thoughts, fostering interoception and supporting present moment awareness.

When teaching prāṇāyāma, consider **pausing at the end of each round** or practice to invite students to notice and sense the effects of the practice on the body, breath and mind. This helps students to be aware of the benefits of the practices and also to assess if it is an appropriate practice for them.

Contraindications and precautions for prāṇāyāma

Sensing and regulating the breath can be immensely helpful for students experiencing mental health challenges, but it can also be triggering and counterproductive if it is not taught sensitively and with **authentic encouragement to adapt or cease the practice at any time**. It is not enough to give lip service to modifications. Teachers need to consistently and compassionately remind their students to tune into their own needs and preferences, and model this behaviour throughout the class.

When teaching prāṇāyāma, **never insist your students close their eyes** as this has the potential to be triggering and feel unsafe, particularly for those experiencing anxiety or trauma. Instead, consider either *inviting* students to choose if they would prefer their eyes open or closed, or simply avoid giving any guidelines about the eyes and students will naturally gravitate towards one or the other.

To reduce the likelihood of an abreaction with any prāṇāyāma practice, I suggest **starting very gently and building up over a period of time**. Keep the focus on the breath being comfortable and easeful, and without force.

Be sure to let your students know that **if they begin to feel uncomfortable or dizzy** they should cease the practice at any time and breathe naturally again. In a group class, it is impossible to know what is going on for all your students and, while in a private session you will probably have more of an idea, you cannot know the full internal experience of your students. So, it is a good idea to preface any prāṇāyāma practice with instructions about what to do if they feel uncomfortable or dizzy, letting them know that prāṇāyāma is designed to be practised in a way that is easeful and comfortable and not forceful or punishing.

While in many prāṇāyāma practices we invite students to close their mouth and **breathe through their nose**, know this will not be comfortable or possible for all of your students. By all means invite your students to breathe through the nose if that is part of the practice, but consider also offering the option to breathe through the mouth with the lips gently parted instead, or breathe in any way that feels natural and comfortable for them. **Natural and comfortable** is much more important than getting the technique *right*.

While some students benefit from the extra sensory feedback of **placing their hands on their abdomen** during abdominal breathing, those experiencing body image concerns or eating disorders may find focusing or placing their hands on their abdomen stressful or triggering. In this case, consider inviting students to place their hands on their ribs instead, or leave out cues to place their hands on their body at all.

As was highlighted in the āsana section, when you are teaching prāṇāyāma, do your best to **avoid sounding controlling**. If we are not careful, prāṇāyāma instructions can sound regimented and controlling, and this may be triggering for people who have had an experience of trauma that involved being controlled. It can also encourage students to override their own instincts about their breath, which is the opposite of what we want to do. Instead, consider using language that is invitational, inclusive, non-judgemental, accurate, fosters connection and encourages curiosity, as we explored in the Therapeutic Skills chapter.

While in some settings you might teach **Ujjāyī Prāṇāyāma** (Ocean Breath) as a means to assist in hearing the breath and to stimulate the vagus nerve, know that doing so has the potential to be triggering for someone with a history of trauma who could either hear their own breathing or the breathing of another during the traumatic experience. So, if you know your student has a history of trauma, or are teaching in a specialized mental health setting, it might be wise to avoid teaching Ujjāyī Prāṇāyāma altogether.

And finally, **keep it simple**, there is rarely a need for complicated techniques.

Meditation

When experiencing depression, anxiety, stress or trauma, it is not uncommon to have a busy and ruminative mind, so **engaging the mind with a guided meditation** practice can be helpful. Many people, when experiencing mental health challenges, have told me that they find unguided or self-directed meditation practices too hard or too triggering, and having someone guide them through the practice can be helpful and make meditation more accessible.

There are many ways to guide your students through meditation, including yoga nidra, progressive muscle relaxation, gratitude, visualizations or self-compassion meditations, counting the breath or any practices that involve guiding students to focus on the breath.

Active meditations can be particularly helpful for students experiencing mental health challenges, as they are often more accessible, do not require you to sit still and can help to shift the focus away from the mind and thoughts. Two of the many ways to practise active meditation include sensing the body during āsana or during a walking meditation practice. Indeed, anything can become a meditation practice: washing the dishes, walking the dog, having a shower, eating dinner or rolling up your yoga mat after class (my favourite!).

I suggest **keeping meditation practices short**, even to just a couple of minutes, particularly for students new to meditation and those with moderate to severe symptoms.

It can also be very helpful to **let students know beforehand how long the practice will be**. It can be easier to tolerate something difficult if we know that it is not going to go on for very long and if we have a clear idea of when it will end. If students do find meditation difficult and they stick at it anyway, they may get the lived experience of doing something challenging and it being okay, which can be helpful in developing distress tolerance. However, this is not something that we necessarily want to encourage our students to do, particularly if you are not a trained mental health professional; instead, it could be an outcome that they naturally experience for themselves in the safe container that you have created.

Contraindications and precautions for meditation

As we have already explored, our minds can get pretty active when we are experiencing mental health challenges. If you do not **give an active mind something to focus on**, it may ruminate, have anxious or depressive thoughts, feel triggered by internal experiences and/or feel restless.

So, if you offer meditation, I suggest **keeping the meditations short and giving the mind something to focus on**, especially at the beginning of class or the beginning of the meditation practice.

Be sure to always **introduce meditation as optional**, so students can choose to opt in or opt out of practising meditation. Remember also that both āsana and prāṇāyāma can be meditation when students are present with their body and breath, so you might choose to not use the 'm' word at all, as some students have had a negative experience with meditation in the past and feel averse to it. Instead, you might weave an active or breath-focused practice into the class that has a meditative quality, but is not a formal seated meditation practice.

As highlighted in the prāṇāyāma section of this chapter, **never insist on eyes being closed** during meditation, as this has the potential to be triggering or feel unsafe. Consider either inviting students to choose if they would prefer their eyes open or closed, or simply avoid giving any guidelines about the eyes and students will naturally gravitate towards one or the other, depending on their preference. Yes, you can practise meditation with the eyes open!

While **visualization meditations** can be helpful for some students, they do have the potential to be triggering. For example, you could guide a meditation with the sound of the ocean in the background, thinking that it would be calming and nourishing, but one of your students may have had a traumatic experience of nearly drowning in the ocean, and this meditation could bring that experience back to the surface. If you are teaching in a specialized mental health setting or if you know your students have a history of trauma, you might avoid guided visualizations or, instead ask your students to share something that they find comforting or nurturing and tailor the guided meditation or soundscape to meet their individual needs.

There has been much discussion about the **shadow side of meditation** for individuals experiencing mental illness,[21] and meditation *can* be harmful if it is not taught appropriately, sensitively and to the needs of the individual. Meditation has the potential to precipitate psychosis, exacerbate obsessive and schizoid traits, and release a debilitating flood of painful emotion in some seriously unwell individuals.[22]

In an article titled 'Meditation and Psychiatry', the author suggests that when sharing meditation with those experiencing mental illness we consider 'to whom, for what symptom, in what form, in what dose, and for how long?'[23] He provides the following information regarding the appropriateness of meditation as an adjunct to psychiatric care:

> The patient must not be psychotic or have too severe a character disorder, so as to avoid any psychiatric complications. Indications for meditation include the treatment of depression, anger, anxiety, stress, hypertension, addiction, insomnia, and chronic pain. Given its effects

> on awareness of self and others, availability and tolerance of affect, and ability to inhibit action, meditation is also a useful practice for patients with neuroses and mild to moderately severe character disorders who are plagued by defensiveness, lack of self-awareness, vulnerability to intense and painful affects, and self-destructive behaviours. If applied intelligently, meditation can help those who are sufficiently motivated to practice.[24]

If you are teaching a group of students experiencing moderate-to-severe mental illness, I suggest avoiding teaching formal meditation unless you are also a trained mental health professional or a yoga therapist experienced in mental health and you have assessed the appropriateness of meditation for the individual. If you have a student in a general yoga class who you know is experiencing moderate-to-severe mental illness, consider speaking to them individually about the appropriateness of meditation for them and offering them other alternatives.

In a general yoga class, if meditation is taught within the guidelines I have suggested above – in a thoughtful and sensitive way, always presented as optional and within a safe and compassionate container – then the likelihood of harm is minimal.

Class plan

Download a yoga class plan for a balanced class at www.mentalhealthawareyoga.com/book-resources.

PRACTICES FOR REDUCING RAJAS

Let us look now at yoga practices and sequences for when rajas is dominant. These can be helpful when our students are hyper-aroused, as we often see in anxiety, trauma and stress.

To *meet our students where they are*, consider starting with more dynamic or energizing practices and gradually, over the course of the class, introducing more calming or down-regulating practices. This might involve starting with a standing āsana sequence that includes movement and flow, then gradually slowing down to seated and less dynamic āsanas, followed by a gentle prāṇāyāma practice and a guided meditation in Śavāsana (Corpse Pose or, as I like to call it if the word 'corpse' does not feel appropriate, 'lying on your back'). We could think of this as a sequence that moves from Tadāsana (Mountain Pose) to Śavāsana.

This principle can be applied to any style of yoga and to the individual needs of your students. For example, the energizing part of a vinyasa flow class will probably look very different than the energizing part of a restorative yoga class; however, in both of these examples, we can begin with a *relatively* more dynamic sequence and gradually slow the class down to a relatively gentler practice.

In the sections below, I will share some ideas for down-regulating āsana, prāṇāyāma and meditation practices that may be helpful when rajas is dominant. All of these suggestions are in addition to those mentioned in the 'Practices for cultivating sattva' section of this chapter and are designed to be tailored to meet the needs of the students in front of you. My hope is that you use these ideas as a springboard for your own creativity in designing classes with your individual students in mind.

Āsana

Consider meeting your rajasic students where they are by beginning with more active āsanas and sequences and gradually transitioning to āsanas and sequences that have a more calming or nourishing effect.

Active practices that may be helpful at the beginning of class for students with a predominance of rajas include:

- dynamic sequences, like Sūrya Namaskar (Sun Salutations) or Marjaryāsana-Bitilāsana (Cat/Cow Sequence)
- moving between āsanas in dynamic and energizing ways, including vinyasas or flowing sequences
- āsanas or variations of āsanas that are more strenuous, for example, Vīrabhadrāsanas (Warrior Poses), Utthita Trikonāsana (Triangle Pose), Vṛkṣāsana (Tree Pose) and Tadāsana (Mountain Pose)
- moving repetitions of postures, instead of long holds.

Calming practices that can be helpful to share towards the end of class for students with a predominance of rajas include:

- moving between āsanas slowly and calmly
- āsanas or variations of āsanas that are more gentle and less strenuous, including seated Ardha Matsyendrāsana variations (Half Lord of the Fishes Poses), Gomukhāsana (Cow Face Pose), Baddha Koṇāsana (Butterfly Pose), Bhūjaṅgāsana (Cobra Pose), Makārāsana (Crocodile Pose) or Supta Matsyendrāsana (Supine Spinal Twist)
- forward bending postures like Uttānāsana (Standing Forward Fold), Prasārita Pādottānāsana (Wide-Legged Forward Bend), Upaviṣṭa Koṇāsana (Wide-Angle Seated Forward Bend), Jānu Śīrṣāsana (Head-to-Knee Pose), Pāśchimottānāsana (Seated Forward Bend) and Bālāsana (Child's Pose)
- restorative postures like Viparita Kāraṇī (Legs-Up-the-Wall Pose), Restorative Ardha Matsyendrāsana (Supported Seated Twist) and Supported Bālāsana (Child's Pose)
- Śavāsana (Corpse Pose) with a folded blanket under the head, a bolster under the knees, blankets over the body and sandbags in the hands.

Contraindications and precautions for āsana

Students with a rajasic dominance will likely benefit from restorative and gentle āsanas; however, it is also likely that they will find them difficult and feel restless or agitated if practised too early in the class. To overcome this, try **meeting your students where they are** (as we explored in the Therapeutic Skills chapter) by starting with more active practices, then gradually slowing the class down to include more calming practices and perhaps ending the class with restorative postures and/or Śavāsana.

Some students who experience anxiety find that a **vigorous āsana practice helps them to burn up their anxious energy**, and they do not want to practise in a gentle or restorative way. While it can be helpful for some people to practise in a vigorous way, if students only practise dynamic āsanas they may end up becoming even more rajasic and never get the embodied experience of relaxation and sattva.

It is important that we listen to and honour our students' needs and desires for their practice; we do not want to presume that we know more about what they need than they do. However, knowing that it is sometimes difficult to see through our own conditioning, we could gently suggest that they try a short, gentle or restorative practice at the end of a vigorous practice and see how it works for them. But never insist, only offer as an invitation.

Prāṇāyāma

Lengthening the exhalation can be a powerful way to down-regulate the nervous system and to cultivate a sense of calm. A longer exhalation is thought to engage the parasympathetic (rest and digest) branch of the autonomic nervous system and a longer inhalation to activate the sympathetic (fight or flight) branch.

Lengthening the exhalation is sometimes called a *vagus nerve hack*, as it is thought to kickstart the calming influences of the parasympathetic branch of the nervous system. The vagus nerve represents the main component of the parasympathetic nervous system and, as it travels a long path from the brain stem down to the abdomen, it is often described as a *wanderer nerve*. The vagus nerve is thought to be a prime candidate in explaining the effects of prāṇāyāma on mental health, physical health and cognitive performance.[25]

I have found that lengthening the exhalation is one of the simplest and most powerful tools we have in our yogic toolbox for reducing anxiety and stress.

Before we start inviting our students to lengthen the exhalation, however, I suggest inviting them to notice and sense the breath just as it is, as outlined in the prāṇāyāma section on 'Practices for cultivating sattva' in this chapter. And then, if you feel like it would benefit your students, invite them to equalize the breath so their inhalations and the exhalations are approximately even in length (Sama Vṛitti Prāṇāyāma). This may be enough for some students, and both can be given as options instead of extending the breath, particularly in a class setting where you are not able to closely monitor all the students.

For students who are comfortable with noticing and equalizing the breath, you might offer one of the many different yoga practices for extending the exhalation, like counting, sounding or chanting. If you have shared a counting practice to equalize the breath, with four counts in and four counts out, as I outlined in the sattva prāṇāyāma section, then you might extend the exhalation by adding an extra count. So you end up with four counts in and five counts out. If students find this comfortable and easeful you could extend the exhalation to six counts.

Bāhya Kumbhaka, or comfortable breath retention after the exhalation, is thought to be helpful for individuals experiencing anxiety,[26] and can be an effective way to slow down the breath even further. If students find it comfortable to extend the exhalation, consider adding the option of holding the breath after the exhalation. I suggest starting by introducing a *pause* after the exhalation and only if this is comfortable, consider introducing counting that includes retention after the exhalation. For example, four counts on the inhalation, four to six counts on the exhalation and then two counts for the breath retention after the exhalation (or longer if appropriate for the student). As always, start small, gradually building up over an extended period of time, and ensure the emphasis is on ease and comfort.

Chandra Bheda Prāṇāyāma, Left Nostril Breathing, is thought to be helpful for reducing anxiety.[27] This is a variation of Nāḍī Sodhana Prāṇāyāma (Alternate Nostril Breathing) that involves inhaling through the left nostril and exhaling through the right, using a mudra with the right hand to direct the airflow. It is often suggested to balance this afterwards with several rounds of Nāḍī Sodhana Prāṇāyāma.

Ujjāyī Prāṇāyāma, or Ocean Breath, is a gentle breath technique that reduces airflow by slightly contracting the glottis and creating an ocean-like sound. Ujjāyī Prāṇāyāma is thought to have a calming effect on the system as a result of slowing down the breath and stimulating the vagus nerve through the vibration made by the resistance created by the vocal cord contraction.[28] When teaching Ujjāyī Prāṇāyāma to students experiencing anxiety, consider inviting them to only make the sound on the exhalation, as anxious students may tend to *pull in* the inhalation which may increase sympathetic dominance and can be activating rather than calming.[29]

Placing a blanket over the body may be nourishing and grounding when rajas is dominant. When teaching prāṇāyāma in a seated position, consider offering a blanket to place over the shoulders or around the lower back. When teaching lying down, consider offering a nourishing head support and a blanket for students to place over their own body.

Contraindications and precautions for prāṇāyāma

While students with a predominance of rajas generally benefit from deepening and slowing down the breath, if a student is very anxious they may find this difficult and may become more anxious if they are unable to do it. Try **meeting your students where they are** by simply listening, noticing or sensing the breath in the body, as we explored in the sattva prāṇāyāma section. This, on its own, can be helpful for students, and often no additional practices are needed.

When teaching most prāṇāyāma practices, **focus on the breath being comfortable and easeful.** If the student tries to force the breath, it will likely be more activating, not calming, thereby having the opposite effect than intended.

I find that when students who are new to prāṇāyāma start to extend the length of the exhalation, they often force the breath out. In this case, it can be helpful to cue students to *slow down* the exhalation, rather than to extend it. This way they are less likely to think that they need to get rid of more air, or push more air out as they exhale, but rather to gently slow down the exhalation so it takes more time to release the breath.

For some students, **focusing on the breath can be triggering.** If this happens, consider stopping your instructions or directions about the breath and instead focus on something else, like the body or music, or try the 5,4,3,2,1 Grounding Practice in the Mental Health Crisis chapter.

While practising **Ujjāyī Prāṇāyāma** (Ocean Breath) can be incredibly helpful for some, it may be triggering for someone with a history of trauma who could either hear their own breathing or the breathing of another during the traumatic experience. If you are teaching in a specialized mental health setting or if you know your student has a history of trauma, consider avoiding teaching Ujjāyī Prāṇāyāma.

If you do teach Ujjāyī Prāṇāyāma, always offer the practice as optional, avoid demonstrating with an exaggerated sounding breath (which could sound like heavy breathing) and encourage students to practise in a way that is soft and barely audible, without any strain or force.

Consider **avoiding Antāra Kumbhaka**, holding the breath after the inhalation, as this can have an activating effect, and **rapid breathing techniques** such as Kapālabhātī (Skull Shining Breath) or Bhastrika Prāṇāyāma (Bellows Breath), as these also have an activating effect and may trigger a panic attack in someone experiencing anxiety.

Meditation

In addition to all the meditation practices I outlined in the sattva section, an active meditation practice that I have found students really resonate with is the **I Am Here meditation**. I learned this from Amy Weintraub, the author of *Yoga for Depression*.[30]

Invite students to stand in a comfortable position, with their legs about hip width apart and the knees softly bent. On the inhalation, imagine the air/prana/energy (pick whichever word will resonate for your students) travelling up through the feet and the body and say silently to yourself, '*I am*'. On the exhalation, imagine the air/prana/energy travelling back down through the body, the feet and down into the centre of the earth and say silently to yourself, '*here*'. Repeat several times.

This active meditation practice can be done sitting or standing but, if it is within the range of my students, I like to teach it while standing initially.

Personally, I find this is a particularly grounding and nourishing practice when I am feeling scattered and not present. It can be a great practice to do yourself before your students arrive for class so you can be fully present with them. Once, when I was teaching the Mental Health Aware Yoga training in Denmark, there were serious bushfires back home in Australia. It was a real challenge to be present at times when things were so difficult at home, and this practice really helped me to be present with myself and my students.

Counting the breath can be a simple and effective way to focus the mind. You might invite your students to count the breath silently backwards from nine to one in their natural breathing rhythm. To reduce rajas, consider inviting your students to *count down* rather than up, as this is thought to have a calming and relaxing effect.

Placing a blanket over the body can feel nourishing and grounding during meditation. When practising meditation in Śavāsana, consider offering a blanket folded under the head, another blanket over the body or abdomen and sandbags in the hands. If practising in a seated position, try offering a blanket over the shoulders or the lower back. Consider also inviting students to organize their own blankets and bolsters. This teaches them how to do it themselves, so they can continue to use the practices outside the yoga class. It is also less likely to be triggering for a student who experienced abuse in bed.

Watch a video of me folding a blanket to create a nourishing head support for students at www.mentalhealthawareyoga.com/book-resources.

Contraindications and precautions for meditation

There are no additional contraindications or precautions for meditation to reduce rajas. Be sure to review the contraindications in the sattva section, as these apply here as well.

Class plan

Download a yoga class plan that focuses on reducing rajas at www.mentalhealthawareyoga.com/book-resources.

PRACTICES FOR REDUCING TAMAS

Let us look now at yoga practices and sequences for when tamas is dominant. These can be helpful when our students are hypo-aroused, as we often see in depression, trauma or low mood.

To meet our students where they are, consider starting with more stable and easeful practices and gradually, over the duration of the class, introducing more energizing or up-regulating practices. This might involve beginning the class lying in Śavāsana and gently moving the head side-to-side or hugging the knees towards the chest, then gradually moving to more dynamic seated and then standing āsanas, threading prāṇāyāma into the movement and ending with a short guided Śavāsana or seated prāṇāyāma practice. We could think of this as a sequence that moves from Śavāsana to Tadāsana.

In the sections below, you will find some ideas for up regulating āsana, prāṇāyāma and meditation practices that may be helpful when tamas is dominant. All of these suggestions are in addition to those mentioned in the sattva section of this chapter and are designed to be customized and personalized to meet the needs of the students in front of you.

Āsana

Consider meeting your tamasic students where they are by beginning with gentle and calming āsanas and sequences and gradually moving to āsanas and sequences with more of an energizing quality.

Gentle or calming practices to share towards the beginning of class for students with a predominance of tamas may include:

- moving between āsanas slowly and calmly
- restorative postures, for example Viparita Kāraṇī (Legs-Up-the-Wall Pose), Restorative Ardha Matsyendrāsana (Supported Seated Twist), Supported Sūpta Baddha Koṇāsana (Reclined Butterfly Pose), Elevated Śavāsana (Corpse Pose with torso elevated on a bolster) and Supported Bālāsana (Child's Pose)
- āsanas or variations of āsanas that may be considered more gentle and less strenuous, including seated Ardha Matsyendrāsana variations (Half Lord of the Fishes Poses), Gomukhāsana (Cow Face Pose), Baddha Koṇāsana (Butterfly Pose), Makārāsana (Crocodile Pose) and Supta Matsyendrāsana (Supine Spinal Twist) .
- forward bending postures, like Bālāsana (Child's Pose), Jānu Śīrṣāsana (Head-to-Knee Pose), Pāśchimottānāsana (Seated

Forward Bend), Upaviṣṭa Koṇāsana (Wide-Angle Seated Forward Bend), Uttānāsana (Standing Forward Fold) and Prasārita Pādottānāsana (Wide-Legged Forward Bend).

Active practices that may be helpful towards the end of class for students with a predominance of tamas may include:

- moving between āsanas in dynamic and energizing ways, including vinyasas or flowing sequences
- dynamic sequences like Marjaryāsana-Bitilāsana (Cat/Cow Sequence) or Sūrya Namaskar (Sun Salutations)
- āsanas or variations of āsanas that are more strenuous, for example, Vīrabhadrāsanas (Warrior Poses), Utthita Trikonāsana (Triangle Pose), Vṛkṣāsana (Tree Pose), Nāvāsana (Boat Pose) and Tadāsana (Mountain Pose).
- chest opening/back bending āsanas, for example, Bhūjaṅgāsana (Cobra Pose), Śalabhasana (Locust Pose), Ūrdhva Mukha Śvānāsana (Upward Facing Dog Pose) and Setu Bandha Sārvaṅgāsana (Bridge Pose)
- moving repetitions of postures rather than long holds.

Contraindications and precautions for āsana

Students with a tamasic dominance generally benefit from more energizing āsanas; however, they may resist or be reluctant to try them. Try **meeting your students where they are** by starting with something gentle, like Bālāsana (Child's Pose) or a gentle Marjaryāsana-Bitilāsana (Cat/Cow) sequence, and gradually make the class more dynamic.

If offering **chest-opening or back-bending practices**, consider also offering a neutral or forward-folding variation, as chest-opening practices have the potential to be triggering and anxiety-inducing, especially if someone is experiencing co-morbid anxiety. If appropriate, you could also offer a counter-posture of a forward-folding āsana, and give students the embodied experience of being open and expansive, then nourished and safe, so they may pendulate between the two.

Sometimes a predominance of tamas is a result of burnout, adrenal fatigue, chronic fatigue, postnatal depletion or chronic illness. In these instances students generally do not need practices that are energizing and up-regulating in nature. Instead, consider offering a balance of gentle movement and relaxation.

Prāṇāyāma

Ujjāyī Prāṇāyāma (Ocean Breath) is featured regularly in the yoga research as a recommended way to reduce depression, anxiety and stress.[31] As outlined in the section on reducing rajas, Ujjāyī Prāṇāyāma is a gentle breath technique that reduces airflow by slightly contracting the glottis, creating an ocean-like sound. It generally has a calming effect on the system but, when practised with the sound on both the exhalation and the inhalation, it may also be mildly activating.

Antāra Kumbhaka, comfortable holding after the inhalation, is thought to be helpful for individuals experiencing depression.[32] If students are able to easily and comfortably regulate the breath, then consider adding the option of holding the breath after the inhalation. Start by introducing a *pause* after the inhalation and, if this is comfortable, consider introducing counting that includes retention after the inhalation. For example, four counts on the inhalation, two counts retention and four counts on the exhalation. As always, start small, gradually building up over an extended period of time, and ensure the emphasis is on ease and comfort.

Gently **lengthening the inhalation** can also have an activating effect and can support energizing the body and mind and reducing tamas. Before we start inviting students to lengthen their inhalation, however, I suggest inviting them to notice and sense the breath just as it is, and then to equalize the breath, as in Sama Vritti Prāṇāyāma, so the inhalations and the exhalations are even (see the sattva prāṇāyāma section for more details). This may be enough for some students, and both can be given as options instead of extending the inhalation, particularly in a class setting where you are not able to closely monitor all your students.

In my experience equalizing the breath is often sufficient and lengthening the inhalation is often not required.

Surya Bheda Prāṇāyāma, Right Nostril Breathing, is another energizing breath practice. It is a variation of Nāḍī Sodhana Prāṇāyāma

(Alternate Nostril Breathing) that involves inhaling through the right nostril and exhaling through the left, using a mudra with the right hand to direct the airflow. It is suggested to balance this by concluding the practice with a few rounds Nāḍī Sodhana Prāṇāyāma.

Sītalī or Sītkalī Prāṇāyāma is thought to have a cooling or calming effect on the mind and to help to regulate the breath and heart rate.[33] With the emphasis on the inhalation, it can have an activating effect.

Kapālabhātī, or Skull Shining Breath, is a kriyā practice (not technically prāṇāyāma) that is thought to be cleansing and energizing, waking up dormant prāṇā if you are feeling depressed.[34] Research has shown that Kapālabhātī increases sympathetic activity in the autonomic nervous system.[35]

Bhastrika Prāṇāyāma, or Bellows Breath, works on the same activating principle as Kapālabhātī and has been found to result in emotional calming and mental alertness afterwards.[36] In Bhastrika Prāṇāyāma, the difference is that the inhalation is deep, forceful and equal to the exhalation, and the pace is usually slower.[37]

Contraindications and precautions for prāṇāyāma

Kapālabhātī and Bhastrika Prāṇāyāma are considered to be advanced breathing techniques, only to be taught by experienced teachers and to students who are ready for the practice. I would not suggest sharing these practices with new students, those who are not proficient at prāṇāyāma, students who you do not know well enough to assess if it is appropriate for them or not or those with co-morbid anxiety.

Be sure to review the contraindications in the sattva section, as these apply here as well.

Meditation

Counting the breath can be a simple and effective way to focus the mind. You might invite your students to count the breath silently from one up to nine in their natural breathing rhythm. To reduce tamas, try *counting up*, rather than down, as this is thought to have an activating effect. Counting up can also be a great idea if you are leading yoga nidra or other relaxing meditations, to support your students to stay awake and alert.

Contraindications and precautions for meditation

There are no additional contraindications or precautions for meditation to reduce tamas. Be sure to review the contraindications in the sattva section, as these apply here as well.

Class plan

Download a yoga class plan that focuses on reducing tamas at www.mentalhealthawareyoga.com/book-resources.

IN THE YOGA CLASS

So, how do we bring everything from this chapter into a yoga class when we have students with different guṇas, presentations and needs?

Excellent question!

Even though many teachers I speak to have concerns about how to sequence a class with students who have a mix of rajasic, tamasic and sattvic presentations, I am often surprised at how similar the energy is among students in a yoga class.

There might be a theme of stress and busy-ness in a class (rajas), a theme of heaviness or sluggishness (tamas), a theme of exhaustion and burnout (tamas after an extended period of rajas) or a theme of clarity and willingness to show up and be present (sattva). When this is the case, it makes sequencing the class much easier, as you can sequence the whole class for reducing tamas or rajas or whatever is required in your particular class.

In a class where all the students are stressed out, anxious, busy or rajasic, you could offer a class that focuses on reducing rajas, starting with more energizing practices and gradually slowing the class down.

When all the students seem heavy, sluggish or depressed you might offer a class that focusses on reducing tamas, starting in a gentle way and gradually becoming more dynamic.

In a class where all the students seem exhausted and burnt out, like in a group of new parents or after a traumatic incident in the area you are teaching in, you might see that, even though your students have a predominance of tamas, they need nurturing and rest; therefore, you might consider offering a class that is deeply nourishing and restorative.

Paradoxically, in this case, offering practices that increase tamas can help students to recover.

If all the students seem relatively sattvic, with a clarity and willingness to show up and be present, you might consider offering them a balanced class, sharing many of the practices from the initial section of this chapter on cultivating sattva.

The challenge comes when there is a mix of rajasic, tamasic and sattvic energies in the class. This is when the teacher draws on their own sattvic wisdom and creativity.

When this happens, I have found that offering a balanced class, with variations for each posture or practice, that either reduce tamas or rajas, depending on how they are practised, can be helpful to meet most people's needs.

Let me share some examples. If you are offering Sūrya Namaskar (Sun Salutations), you might invite students who are feeling sluggish the opportunity to energize by doing an extra round of Sūrya Namaskar; and, for those who are feeling stressed or anxious, you might offer the opportunity to calm their nervous system by resting into Bālāsana (Child's Pose) during the final round, noticing the movement of the breath in their belly as they breathe in and out.

In Vīrabhadrāsana A (Warrior Pose A), you could invite your students to place their back knee on the mat and hands on the ground for a more gentle or nourishing variation, or invite them to straighten the back leg and lift the body and arms up for a more energizing or active variation.

In a prone position, you could invite students to rest in Makārāsana (Crocodile Pose) for a more calming or nourishing variation, or to lift their upper body into Bhujaṅgāsana (Cobra Pose) or into Urdhvamukha Svānāsana (Upward-Facing Dog) for a relatively more energizing variation. Usually, we offer these variations based on a student's abilities, but we can also offer them based on a continuum of calming to energizing.

In Balāsana (Child's Pose), you might suggest students extend their arms and rest up on their fingertips for a more energizing version of the practice, or soften their arms down onto the floor, or lie their arms by their sides for a more nourishing or calming variation. This can be a particularly helpful variation as students are face down and cannot see easily what the other students are choosing. In addition, they are unlikely to have a value judgement about which variation is *better* or *more advanced*, so have the opportunity to make a decision based on what they need rather than what they *think* is the best option.

If you are offering a restorative posture, you may offer the variation of Supported Supta Baddha Konāsana (Reclined Butterfly Pose) for those who are needing a slightly more energizing practice and Supported Balāsana (with the bolster under the chest and abdomen) for those who are looking for a more calming and nourishing practice. While we may not usually think about Supported Supta Baddha Konāsana as an energizing practice, it could be argued that is relatively more energizing than Supported Balāsana.

I find it helpful to support your students to make wise choices for themselves by mentioning who the variation may be for, for example, those needing more energizing or calming practices. Otherwise, tamasic students may naturally choose the variation that increases tamas, and rajasic students may naturally choose the variation that increases rajas.

There are endless ways of offering different variations of practices and postures, and we want to do what we can to support our students to find the best variation for them. Be creative and experiment in your classes, and find ways that work best for you and your students. This is where the fun and magic happen!

Class plan

Download a yoga class plan for a balanced or mixed class at www.mentalhealthawareyoga.com/book-resources.

COMPASSIONATE REFLECTION

1. Which of these practices or sequences are you already integrating into your yoga teaching?

2. Were there any new practices or new ways of sharing practices in this chapter that you would like to bring into your teaching to support the mental health of your students?

3. Try one of these out, then spend some time reflecting on how it went, including what went well, what did not go so well and what you would do differently next time.

Pillar Six

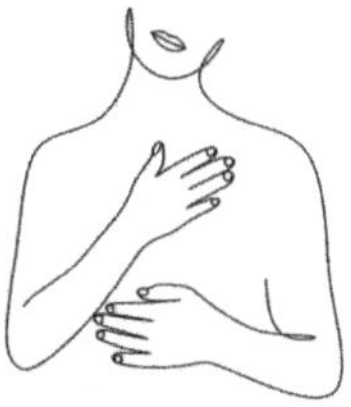

MENTAL HEALTH CRISIS

Do you know what to do if a student in your class cries, becomes anxious or overwhelmed or has a panic attack?

I believe that it is important for all humans to know how to support each other in times of distress. With nearly 80% of yoga students reporting that they practise yoga for mental health reasons,[1] it is particularly important for yoga teachers.

While creating a safe container and teaching practices that address the needs of the individual student can help to reduce the likelihood of anxiety, overwhelm, dysregulation and panic occurring, we cannot prevent these from happening. And sometimes it is only *when* we feel safe, like many of our students do in our yoga classes, that suppressed emotion bubbles up to the surface and we may find our students crying on the mat.

CRYING

Emily went to a yoga class not long after the death of her mother and found herself crying in class, something she would normally never do. Emily had a very demanding job, managing the physiotherapy department of a large hospital and raising two young children and, after her mother's funeral, she found that she was too busy to grieve. But in the safe space of her regular yoga class with a teacher she trusted, and with nothing to do but be present with herself, the tears flowed.

Emily was not in crisis. The teacher did not do anything wrong to cause the tears to come. Rather the safe space and the gentle time to be present with herself meant that she was finally able to feel the things she had been too busy to feel, and she began the process of healthy grieving.

Emily is not the only one who has experienced something like this. Perhaps you have cried in a yoga class too? I know I have!

Reacting to crying

When someone cries in our presence it can bring up our own unresolved emotion, and we can find it difficult to cope. When this happens, it can go a few different ways.

We might back away or ignore the person who is crying and pretend that it is not happening. If we do not see it, then we do not have to address it!

We might try to shut down the emotion in the other person, in one of a multitude of different ways, like telling them that it is going to be okay, distracting them with something else, giving them a yoga practice to stop the crying or by changing the subject.

Or perhaps we swoop in and try to help, to fix the problem and make everything better (aka the *rescuer)*, as we explored in the Safe Container chapter.

All of these responses are usually attempts to regulate our *own* internal experience and, while they usually come from a well-meaning place, they are rarely helpful and often everyone involved is left feeling a little off kilter.

To overcome this, we need to learn to sit in our own emotions and to allow ourselves to cry when we need to. If we cannot allow ourselves to cry, it is very difficult to be present with someone else when they are crying.

Equally, we need to address our own beliefs about helping and rescuing and trust that our students are able to cry and still be safe and okay, that there is nothing that we need to fix.

Crying is not actually a mental health crisis, it is usually a very healthy response to life's challenges, but, if we are not equipped to deal with it, it can feel like a crisis.

Responding to crying

I have found that, in most situations, the best thing to do when someone cries in a yoga class is to simply let them cry, and sensitively and compassionately let them know that you see them.

When we back away or ignore crying or when we try to stop it or shut it down, even in a well-meaning way, we are communicating that crying is shameful or that it is not okay.

If a student cries in class, instead of saying, 'it's okay' or 'there, there don't cry' and stepping in for an unasked for hug, try quietly and respectfully acknowledging that you have seen them crying and are available if they need you, and discreetly check in with them after class.

If your student still appears to be upset or is crying at the end of class, consider checking in with them to see if they have someone to support them after class, like a friend, a family member or a therapist they can call.

Remember to stay within your scope of practice and compassionately watch for any rescuer behaviour in yourself (as we explored in the Safe Container chapter).

If you notice that you are triggered by someone crying in your class, this could be an invitation for you to do some self-enquiry in meditation, in your journal, with a trusted friend or with a therapist.

ANXIETY AND OVERWHELM

Even in the most calming of yoga classes, with an experienced, warm and skilful teacher, students can still experience anxiety or overwhelm.

Attending a yoga class can feel way outside the comfort zone of many people. Yoga studios often look different to many other places people have been to before; people are dressed differently, the teacher and/or other students might be unfamiliar, the language is often new and strange, the positions that students are often asked to place their bodies in can be unusual, the room can feel too full or too stuffy if the windows are not open, and students might be concerned that they do not look like they fit in or worry that they will not know what to do and will stand out.

It can be a world of uncertainty and self-doubt!

Some of the postures and practices of yoga also have the potential to trigger anxiety, including chest opening or back bending postures, prāṇāyāma practices with rapid breathing or calming postures that the student feels unable to do as their mind is racing and their heart is beating fast.

In addition, a student with a history of trauma may be triggered by something in class, and, as a result, experience fear, flashbacks, dissociation or disconnection.

Students with a lived experience of anxiety or trauma may be more likely to experience heightened anxiety or overwhelm in a yoga class. As a result, it is important to be mindful of the potential for this and do our best to create a safe container and share practices (or variations of practices) to meet the needs of students experiencing anxiety and trauma (see the Yogic Practices chapter for suggestions).

However, we do not need to become anxious ourselves about preventing our students from feeling anxiety or being triggered. By holding a safe container, we create a space where students may safely meet their anxiety. While we would never wish to create an anxiety-inducing experience, anxiety showing up in a yoga class can be an opportunity for students to meet and move through their anxiety, if they feel safe and supported.

Responding to anxiety

One of the most helpful things you can do if a student in your class appears anxious, overwhelmed or triggered is to stay calm yourself, and do your best to exude a warm and welcoming presence. This can help to communicate that you are not concerned about them feeling anxious, that anxiety is welcome in the yoga class, that you are not judging them, that you trust that they can meet whatever arises within them and that you are available for support, if needed.

Staying calm yourself can also engage the mirror neuron system and may help to foster a sense of calm.

Consider also discreetly checking in with them at the end of class and, if needed, ask if they have someone to support them afterwards, like a friend, a family member or a therapist.

Be supportive, stay within your scope of practice and compassionately watch for any rescuer behaviour.

PANIC ATTACKS

A panic attack is a discrete episode of intense anxiety. The experience is usually very distressing and physically uncomfortable. Many people report that they feel like they are having a heart attack or that they are going to die, especially if it is the first time they have experienced a panic attack or if they do not understand what is happening. A panic attack can be very scary, but it is not life threatening or dangerous.

Panic and yoga

In a yoga class, a student may experience a panic attack if they feel very unsafe.

If the exit is blocked (for example by another student practising in front of the door) or if the door is locked from the inside (for example to prevent late students from entering), a student might feel like they cannot leave if they need to, and this could cause anxiety or panic. I have heard from teachers who live in countries where gun violence is an everyday reality that students can feel also unsafe if the door is *un*locked.

Other reasons why a student might feel unsafe and experience panic include if a student does not know if the teacher is going to touch them or single them out in front of the class, if they are asked to do partner work that they are not comfortable with or if the lights are turned off during Śavāsana (Corpse Pose).

We can reduce the likelihood of this occurring by doing what we can to create a safe space to teach in as we explored in Safe Container chapter.

A panic attack could also occur as a result of a yoga practice. Students may feel light-headed, out of breath or uncomfortable in a practice, particularly a practice involving rapid breathing like Kapālabhātī Prāṇāyāma (Skull Shining Breath), breath retention after the inhalation, or even with chest opening or back-bending practices. These could induce a panic attack, particularly if someone is currently experiencing or has a history of anxiety, panic or trauma.

I suggest not offering these practices to students who you know experience anxiety or panic, particularly if you are not a mental health professional who can use their clinical judgement to assess if it is appropriate for the individual and can support the student if they have an abreaction.

If you do offer these practices to a group of students, always assume that there might be someone experiencing or with a history of anxiety or panic in the group, and let the class know that these practices are contraindicated for anxiety and offer other alternatives.

In meditation, a student could be triggered by a visualization or an internal experience, such as an emotion, thought, memory or image. When you are teaching meditation, I suggest always giving your students the option to practise with their eyes open or closed, letting them know that they are in the driver's seat and can stop listening to your voice at any time or open their eyes whenever they like, supporting them to cultivate inner and outer resources.

If a student has had a traumatic experience (including a previous panic attack), there could be something about the class that triggers the memory and leads to anxiety or panic. Perhaps there is someone in the class that reminds them of someone else, the smell of the room or the smell of the deodorant of another student, the light coming through the windows in a certain way, someone yelling outside the class or being in a group of people in an enclosed space.

While we may do everything we can to create a safe container and choose appropriate practices and variations, we cannot control all the variables, as we do not know everyone's history or their current state. If a student does have a panic attack, however, we can support them through it.

What to do if someone has a panic attack

If you believe someone is having a panic attack, remain calm yourself and speak to them in a warm and reassuring manner. Ask them if they have ever experienced a panic attack before, and if there is anything you can do to help. If you are not sure if they are having a panic attack or not, especially if they have never had a panic attack before, or they lose consciousness, call for help and follow first aid guidelines.

One way to support a student if they are feeling anxious or panicked is to invite them to join you for a 5,4,3,2,1 Grounding Practice. If it is appropriate, consider inviting the student (or the whole class) to notice five things that they can see, four things they can feel, three things they can hear, two things they can smell (or enjoy smelling) and one thing they can taste, pausing in between each sense and inviting them to state the sense objects either silently or aloud. Attending to the present moment through the senses may help students to bring themselves into the present moment by noticing the sensory experience of their environment.

Watch a video of me sharing this practice at www.mentalhealthawareyoga.com/book-resources.

Be sure to always stay within your scope of practice and consider referring the student to someone who has experience with panic attacks, like a psychologist or other mental health professional.

We go into much more detail about supporting someone experiencing a mental health crisis in the Mental Health Aware Yoga training, but the information here is a great place to start.

COMPASSIONATE REFLECTION

1. Have you ever cried, felt overwhelmed or anxious, or had a panic attack? What happened?
2. What was unhelpful in this situation?
3. What was helpful?
4. What would you have liked to have happened?
5. Has a student ever cried, felt overwhelmed or anxious, or had a panic attack in one of your classes?
6. How did you respond?
7. If it happened again, what would you do?

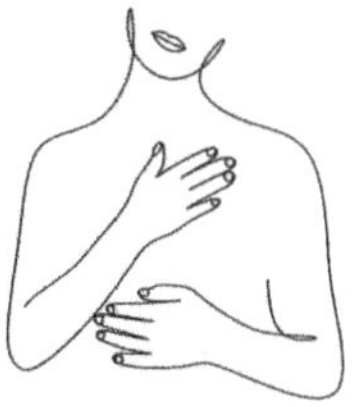

WHERE TO FROM HERE

Thank you for reading all the way to the end of the book! Honestly, it warms my heart to think about you reading through these pages and bringing these ideas into your teaching and into your life.

It took me far too long to integrate and embody what I read in yoga books into my life and work, and my hope for you is that you do not take as long as I did (although if you do, know that you are in good company)! Intellectual understanding is a great start, but it is not enough on its own. To really understand this work, we need to *do* the practices and *live* the teachings.

So, my invitation to you, should you choose to accept it, is to choose just *one* idea from this book and try it out. Just one! There is a lot of information and ideas within these pages, and I know how overwhelming that can be. But what if you picked just one thing and tried it out in your own life or in your yoga teaching?

Then, afterwards, consider taking some time to reflect on the questions: What went well? What didn't go so well? How would I refine it for next time?

And continue this process for as long as you like; reading, practising, reflecting and refining. Really, it is a life pursuit!

You can download all the free resources mentioned throughout this book at www.mentalhealthawareyoga.com/book-resources.

If you feel called (and I hope that you do), I wholeheartedly welcome you to join us for the Mental Health Aware Yoga training. It would be a joy to meet you, either online or in person, and continue this journey together.

In the Mental Health Aware Yoga training we dive even deeper into this work, to lift it off the page and into your life and into your teaching.

You can find all the details at www.mentalhealthawareyoga.com.

Thank you for being here and being part of this evolution of yoga to meet our contemporary needs.

See you on the mat!

Acknowledgements

This book is a long-held dream come true. As long as I can remember, I have been reading and collecting books and harbouring a secret desire to one day see my own book on the shelf in my favourite bookshops. And now you are holding it in your hands!

When Sarah Hamlin from Singing Dragon reached out after hearing my interview on the Connected Yoga Teachers' Podcast and asked me if I would consider submitting a proposal for a book on yoga and mental health, I could hardly believe it. And, of course, the answer was *yes*. In fact, I had already written the first draft.

I wrote the majority of this book on Bundjalung country in Australia, and I am deeply grateful for this land and for its traditional custodians, the Arakwal people. This is my favourite place in the world, and I am grateful to call it home.

I am so grateful to Annabel McLisky, who explored many of the topics I cover in this book with me during the many long drives back and forth from Byron to the Gold Coast. Annabel was one of the first people to read over the initial Mental Health Aware Yoga training manual and was kind enough to give me feedback on this book during a holiday to Italy (thank goodness for long-haul flights). I am also grateful for the wonderful Anneke Sips (let's have that cup of sattvic tea soon) and Sarah Truman (thank you for your enthusiasm for the Mental Health Aware Yoga training) for offering timely feedback on the pages you hold in front of you, and to Candida Baker for helping me navigate the world of publishing. Also, to Kate Reed, who alleviated my anxiety about the permanency of publishing my ideas on paper, and encouraged me to speak to this in the early part of the book. Thank you to Sarah, Jenny, Carys and Sandra from Singing Dragon for your care and belief in bringing this book into the world.

I am deeply grateful for the wisdom of Saraswathi Vasudevan, Ganesh Mohan, Richard Miller and Amy Weintraub for my growing understanding of yoga and mental health over the past few decades. Saraswathi Vasudevan, in particular, provided feedback on the Yoga Psychology section of the Mental Health Aware Yoga training and answered my detailed questions on Patañjali's Yoga Sūtras. I have studied and practised with many teachers over the years, and I thank them and their teachers, and their teachers before them, and all who have passed on the sacred and practical wisdom of yoga.

I am also so grateful for all the compassionate and heart-centred yoga teachers who have joined me for the Mental Health Aware Yoga training and who have helped me to refine my understanding and my ability to communicate many of the ideas that you have read about in this book. They are shining their lights so brightly in their communities, supporting the mental health of their yoga students with such dedication and care. And to the amazing humans who have been working with me at the Yoga Psychology Institute over the past few years, including Stefan, Annabel, Sandra, Zsa Zsa, Jel, Kass, Mich, Ricardo and Trixie. Thank you for your belief in this work and for the support you offer our students.

Sending so much love to Nick, who tragically died while I was editing the final draft of this book, and so is interwoven, along with my tears, into these words. And to Belle, Mai and Oscar. I have no words to describe your loss, but seeing the way you are so loved and supported by your community during this time has given me so much hope for humanity. You are all forever in my heart.

And last, but certainly not least, a big big thank you to Stefan, my husband, who has been unwavering in his support of this work, and our brilliant, noisy and wonderful children, Lukas and Zaia. You all mean the world to me, and I thank you for being exactly who you are, for giving me time and space to write and, yes, I'm coming upstairs now to hang out with you and play with our new puppy, Alviss.

Endnotes

INTRODUCTION

1 Penman, S., Cohen, M., Stevens, P. & Jackson, S. (2012). Yoga in Australia: Results of a National Survey. *International Journal of Yoga, 5(2)*, 92–101.

2 Australian Bureau of Statistics. (2007). *National Survey of Mental Health and Wellbeing: Summary of Results, Australia, 2007.* ABS cat. no. 4326.0. Canberra: ABS.

3 Mental Health Foundation. (2016). *Fundamental Facts About Mental Health 2016.* London: Mental Health Foundation.

4 Kessler R. C., Berglund P., Demler O., Jin R., Merikangas K. R. & Walters E. E. (2005). Lifetime Prevalence and Age-of-Onset Distributions of DSM-IV Disorders in the National Comorbidity Survey Replication. *Archives of General Psychiatry, 62*, 593–602.

5 Australian Bureau of Statistics. (2007). *National Survey of Mental Health and Wellbeing: Summary of Results, Australia, 2007.* ABS cat. no. 4326.0. Canberra: ABS.

6 Global Burden of Disease Study 2013 Collaborators. (2015). Global, Regional, and National Incidence, Prevalence, and Years Lived with Disability for 301 Acute and Chronic Diseases and Injuries in 188 Countries, 1990–2013: A Systematic Analysis for the Global Burden of Disease Study 2013. *Lancet (London, England), 386(9995)*, 743–800.

7 Penman, S., Cohen, M., Stevens, P., & Jackson, S. (2012). Yoga in Australia: Results of a National Survey. *International Journal of Yoga, 5(2)*, 92–101.

8 Egan, G. (2002). *The Skilled Helper.* Pacific Grove, CA: Brooks/Cole.

PILLAR ONE

1 American Psychiatric Association. (2013). *Diagnostic and Statistical Manual of Mental Disorders (5th ed.).* Washington, DC: APA.

2 Australian Bureau of Statistics. (2007). *National Survey of Mental Health and Wellbeing: Summary of Results, Australia, 2007.* ABS cat. no. 4326.0. Canberra: ABS.

3 Andrews, G., Creamer, M., Crino, R., Hunt, C., Lampe, L. & Page, A. (2003). *The Treatment of Anxiety Disorders.* Cambridge: Cambridge University Press.

4 Australian Bureau of Statistics. (2007). *National Survey of Mental Health and Wellbeing: Summary of Results, Australia, 2007.* ABS cat. no. 4326.0. Canberra: ABS.

5 American Psychiatric Association. (2013). *Diagnostic and Statistical Manual of Mental Disorders (5th ed.).* Washington, DC: APA (pp. 208–9).

6 Herman, J. (1997). *Trauma and Recovery.* New York: Basic Books.

7 van der Kolk, B. (2014). *The Body Keeps the Score.* New York: Viking.

8 Kessler, R. C., Hughes, M., Sonnega, S. & Nelson, C. B. (1995). Posttraumatic Stress Disorder in the National Comorbidity Survey. *Archives of General Psychiatry, 52(12)*, 1048–60.

9 Floen, S. K. & Elklit, A. (2007). Psychiatric Diagnoses, Trauma, and Suicidiality. *Annals of General Psychiatry,* 6, 12.

10 Kessler, R. C., Hughes, M., Sonnega, S. & Nelson, C. B. (1995). Posttraumatic Stress Disorder in the National Comorbidity Survey. *Archives of General Psychiatry, 52(12)*, 1048–60.

11 Australian Bureau of Statistics. (2007). *National Survey of Mental Health and Wellbeing: Summary of Results, Australia.* ABS cat. no. 4326.0. Canberra: ABS.

12 American Psychiatric Association. (2013). *Diagnostic and Statistical Manual of Mental Disorders (5th ed.).* Washington, DC: APA.

13 American Psychiatric Association. (2013). *Diagnostic and Statistical Manual of Mental Disorders (5th ed.).* Washington, DC: APA (pp. 271–4).

14 American Psychiatric Association. (2013). *Diagnostic and Statistical Manual of Mental Disorders (5th ed.).* Washington, DC: APA (pp. 271–4).

15 van der Kolk, B. (2015). Mind, Brain, and Body in the Healing of Trauma. Clinician Workshop in Brisbane, Australia.

16 Herman, J. (1997). *Trauma and Recovery.* New York: Basic Books.

17 Herman, J. (1997). *Trauma and Recovery.* New York: Basic Books (p.121).

18 Herman, J. (1997). *Trauma and Recovery.* New York: Basic Books (p.121).

19 Herman, J. (1997). *Trauma and Recovery.* New York: Basic Books.

20 Nicki, A. (2016). Borderline Personality Disorder, Discrimination, and Survivors of Chronic Childhood Trauma. *International Journal of Feminist Approaches to Bioethics, 9(1)*, 218–45.

21 Australian Psychological Society. (2015). *Stress & Wellbeing: How Australians Are Coping with Life.* https://psychology.org.au/getmedia/ae32e645-a4f0-4f7c-b3ce-dfd83237c281/stress-wellbeing-survey.pdf.

22 Harvard Health Publishing. (2020). *Understanding the Stress Response.* www.health.harvard.edu/staying-healthy/understanding-the-stress-response.

23 Pfeiffer, R. F. (2007). Neurology of Gastroenterology and Herpetology. In *Neurology and Clinical Neuroscience,* ed. A. Schapira. New York: Elsevier (Chapter 114, pp. 1511–24).

24 Million, M. & Larauche, M. (2016). Stress, Sex and the Enteric Nervous System. *Neurogastroenterology and Motility: The Official Journal of the European Gastrointestinal Motility Society, 28(9)*, 1283–9.

25 Yerkes, R. M. & Dodson, J. D. (1908). The Relation of Strength of Stimulus to Rapidity of Habit-Formation. *Journal of Comparative Neurology and Psychology, 18*, 459–82.

26. Diamond, D.M. (2005). Cognitive, Endocrine and Mechanistic Perspectives on Non-Linear Relationships Between Arousal and Brain Function. *Nonlinearity in Biology, Toxicology, and Medicine*, 3, 1–7.

27 Yeung, A. S., Ivkovic, A. & Fricchione, G. L. (2016). *The Science of Stress.* Chicago: The University of Chicago Press.

28 Lamers, F., van Oppen, P., Comijs, H. C., Smit, J. H., *et al.* (2011). Comorbidity Patterns of Anxiety and Depressive Disorders in a Large Cohort Study: The Netherlands Study of Depression and Anxiety (NESDA). *Journal of Clinical Psychiatry, 72(3)*, 341–8.

29 Lamers, F., van Oppen, P., Comijs, H. C., Smit, J. H., *et al.* (2011). Comorbidity Patterns of Anxiety and Depressive Disorders in a Large Cohort Study: The Netherlands Study of Depression and Anxiety (NESDA). *Journal of Clinical Psychiatry, 72(3)*, 341–8.

30 Shah, R., Shah, A. & Links, P. (2012). Post-traumatic Stress Disorder and Depression Comorbidity: Severity Across Different Populations. *Neuropsychiatry, 2(6)*, 521–9.

PILLAR TWO

1 Desikachar, T.K.V. (1995). *The Heart of Yoga.* Rochester, VT: Inner Traditions International.

2 Desikachar, T.K.V. (1995). *The Heart of Yoga.* Rochester, VT: Inner Traditions International.

3 Desikachar, T.K.V. (1995). *The Heart of Yoga.* Rochester, VT: Inner Traditions International (p. 149).

4 Iyengar, B.K.S. (2002). *Light on the Yoga Sūtras of Patañjali.* London: Thorsons (p. 50).

5 Bryant, E. (2009). *The Yoga Sūtras of Patañjali.* New York: North Point Press (p. 10).

6 Feuerstein, G. (2002). *The Yoga Tradition.* Delhi: Bhavana Books and Prints (p. 286).

7 Mehrotra, A. (2019). *This Is That: Patanjali's Yoga Sutras Pada 1 and 2.* Rishikesh: Sattva Publications (p. 16).

8 Barkataki, S. (2020). *Embrace Yoga's Roots: Courageous Ways to Deepen Your Yoga Practice.* Orlando, FL: Ignite Yoga and Wellness Institute (p. 3).

9 Miller, R. (2013). *Level 1 Training Integrative Restoration* (version 4.6c). San Rafael, CA: Anahata Press (p. xxiii).

10 Feuerstein, G. (2002). *The Yoga Tradition.* Delhi: Bhavana Books and Prints.

11 Miller, R. (2012). *The Samkhya Karika.* San Rafael, CA: Anahata Press.

12 Barkataki, S. (2020). *Embrace Yoga's Roots: Courageous Ways to Deepen Your Yoga Practice.* Orlando, FL: Ignite Yoga and Wellness Institute.

13 Miller, R. (2012). *The Samkhya Karika.* San Rafael, CA: Anahata Press.

14 Feuerstein, G. (2002). *The Yoga Tradition.* Delhi: Bhavana Books and Prints (p. 311).

15 Bryant, E. (2009). *The Yoga Sūtras of Patañjali.* New York: North Point Press (pp. 241–2).

16 Bryant, E. (2009). *The Yoga Sūtras of Patañjali.* New York: North Point Press (p. 242).

17 Bryant, E. (2009). *The Yoga Sūtras of Patañjali.* New York: North Point Press.

18 Desikachar, T.K.V. (1995). *The Heart of Yoga.* Rochester, VT: Inner Traditions International.

19 Iyengar, B.K.S. (2000). *Light on Aṣṭāṅga Yoga.* Mumbai: Tata Press.

20 Desikachar, T.K.V. (1995). *The Heart of Yoga.* Rochester, VT: Inner Traditions International.

21 Barataki, S. (2023). Issue #3 Asteya. Yoga Class Curator. Programme attended by author in 2023.

22 Mehrotra, A. (2019). *This Is That: Patanjali's Yoga Sutras Pada 1 and 2.* Rishikesh: Sattva Publications.

23 Desikachar, T.K.V. (1995). *The Heart of Yoga.* Rochester, VT: Inner Traditions International (p. 99).

24 Barataki, S. Issue #4 Brahmacarya. Yoga Class Curator. Programme attended by author in 2023.

25 Bryant, E. (2009). *The Yoga Sūtras of Patañjali.* New York: North Point Press (p. 252).

26 Desikachar, T.K.V. (1995). *The Heart of Yoga.* Rochester, VT: Inner Traditions International.

27 Bryant, Edward. (2009). *The Yoga Sūtras of Patañjali.* New York: North Point Press (p. 253).

28 Emmons, R.A. & McCullough, M. E. (2003). Counting Blessings vs Burdens: An Experimental Investigation of Gratitude and Subjective Well-Being in Daily Life. *Journal of Personality and Social Psychology, 84(2),* 377–89.

29 Rash, J. A., Matsuba, M. K. & Prkachin, K.M. (2011). Gratitude and Wellbeing: Who Benefits the Most from a Gratitude Intervention. *Applied Psychology: Health and Well-Being, 3(3),* 350–69.

30 Feuerstein, G. (2002). *The Yoga Tradition.* Delhi: Bhavana Books and Prints (p. 328).

31 Desikachar, T.K.V. (1995). *The Heart of Yoga.* Rochester, VT: Inner Traditions International (p. 102).

32 Mehrotra, A. (2019). *This Is That: Patanjali's Yoga Sutras Pada 1 and 2.* Rishikesh: Sattva Publications.

33 Barataki, S. Issue #8 Tapas. Yoga Class Curator. Programme attended by author in 2023.

34 Desikachar, T.K.V. (1995). *The Heart of Yoga.* Rochester, VT: Inner Traditions International.

35 Barataki, S. (2023). Discussion with Susanna in Yoga Course Curator Office Hours, 13 April 2023.

36 Bryant, E. (2009). *The Yoga Sūtras of Patañjali.* New York: North Point Press.

37 Vasudevan, S. (2019). Personal communication.

38 Vasudevan, S. (2018). Sutras and Sadhana: The Psychology of Yoga. Seminar in Byron Bay, Australia.

39 Desikachar, T.K.V. (1995). *The Heart of Yoga.* Rochester, VT: Inner Traditions International (pp. 53–69).

40 Vasudevan, S. (2018). Sutras and Sadhana: The Psychology of Yoga. Seminar in Byron Bay, Australia.

41 Desikachar, T.K.V. (1995). *The Heart of Yoga.* Rochester, VT: Inner Traditions International (p. 107).
42 Desikachar, T.K.V. (1995). *The Heart of Yoga.* Rochester, VT: Inner Traditions International.
43 Vasudevan, S. (2018). Sutras and Sadhana: The Psychology of Yoga. Seminar in Byron Bay, Australia.
44 Desikachar, T.K.V. (1998). *Health, Healing and Beyond.* New York: North Point Press.
45 Desikachar, T.K.V. (1995). *The Heart of Yoga.* Rochester, VT: Inner Traditions International.
46 Desikachar, T.K.V. (1995). *The Heart of Yoga.* Rochester, VT: Inner Traditions International.
47 Desikachar, T.K.V. (1995). *The Heart of Yoga.* Rochester, VT: Inner Traditions International.
48 Desikachar, T.K.V. (1995). *The Heart of Yoga.* Rochester, VT: Inner Traditions International.
49 Miller, R. (2012). *The Sāṅkhya Kārikā.* Version 1.3. eBook. Integrative Restoration Institute, www.irest.us.
50 Bryant, E. (2009). *The Yoga Sūtras of Patañjali.* New York: North Point Press.
51 Puta, M. & Sedlmeier, P. (2014). The Concept of Tri-Guna: A Working Model. In *Meditation – Neuroscientific Approaches and Philosophical Implications,* ed. S. Schmidt & H. Walach. Berlin: Springer (pp. 317–64).
52 Siegel, D. J. (2020). *The Developing Mind: How Relations and the Brain Interact to Shape Who We Are (3rd ed.).* New York: Guilford Press (Chapter 7).
53 Desikachar, T.K.V. (1995). *The Heart of Yoga.* Rochester, VT: Inner Traditions International.
54 Sedlmeier, P. & Srinivas, K. (2016). How Do Theories of Cognition and Consciousness in Ancient Indian Thought Systems Relate to Current Western Theorizing and Research? *Frontiers in Psychology, 7,* 343.
55 Vasudevan, S. (2018). Sutras and Sadhana: The Psychology of Yoga. Seminar in Byron Bay, Australia.

PILLAR THREE

1 Cramer, H. & Weintraub, A. (2018). Depression. In *Yoga for Mental Health,* ed. H. Mason and K. Birch. Pencaitland, Scotland: Handspring Publishing.
2 Emerson, D. & Hopper, Elizabeth. (2011). *Overcoming Trauma Through Yoga.* Berkeley, CA: North Atlantic Books.
3 Vasudevan, S. (2018). Sutras and Sadhana: The Psychology of Yoga. Seminar in Byron Bay, Australia.
4 Yoga Australia. *Scope of Practice.* https://yogaaustralia.org.au/advocacy.
5 Mohan, A. G. (2010). *Krishnamacharya: His Life and Teachings.* Boston: Shambhala Publications.
6 Mohan, A. G. (2010). *Krishnamacharya: His Life and Teachings.* Boston: Shambhala Publications (p. 46).

PILLAR FOUR

1 Lim, M. H. (2018). Is Loneliness Australia's Next Public Health Epidemic? *InPsych, 40(4),* 6–11.
2 Emerson, D. & Hopper, E. (2011). *Overcoming Trauma Through Yoga.* Berkeley, CA: North Atlantic Books.
3 van der Kolk, B. (2014). *The Body Keeps the Score.* New York: Viking.
4 Emerson, D. & Hopper, E. (2011). *Overcoming Trauma Through Yoga.* Berkeley, CA: North Atlantic Books.
5 Forbes, B. (2015). Interoception: Mindfulness in the Body. *LA Yoga.* http://boforbes.com/wp-content/uploads/2015/08/MayLAYoga_Page56.pdf.
6 Valenzuela-Moguillansky, C., Reyes-Reyes, A. & Gaete, M. I. (2017). Exteroceptive and Interoceptive Body-Self Awareness in Fibromyalgia Patients. *Frontiers in Human Neuroscience, 11,* 117.
7 Forbes, B. (2015). Interoception: Mindfulness in the Body. *LA Yoga.* http://boforbes.com/wp-content/uploads/2015/08/MayLAYoga_Page56.pdf.

8 Farb, N., Daubenmier, J., Price, C., Gard, T., *et al.* (2015). Interoception, Contemplative Practice, and Health. *Frontiers in Psychology, 6.*

9 van der Kolk, B. (2014). *The Body Keeps the Score.* New York: Viking (p. 273).

PILLAR FIVE

1 Büssing, A., Michalsen, A., Khalsa, S.B.S., Telles, S. & Sherman, K. J. (2012). Effects of Yoga on Mental and Physical Health: A Short Summary of Reviews. *Evidence-based Complementary and Alternative Medicine, 2,* 1–7.

2 Jeter, P. E., Slutsky, J., Singh, N. & Khalsa, S. B. (2015). Yoga as a Therapeutic Intervention: A Bibliometric Analysis of Published Research Studies from 1967 to 2013. *Journal of Alternative and Complementary Medicine, 21(10),* 586–92.

3 Sedlmeier, P. & Srinivas, K. (2016). How Do Theories of Cognition and Consciousness in Ancient Indian Thought Systems Relate to Current Western Theorizing and Research? *Frontiers in Psychology, 7,* 343.

4 Siegel, D. J. (2020). *The Developing Mind: How Relations and the Brain Interact to Shape Who We Are (3rd ed.).* New York: Guilford Press (Chapter 7).

5 van der Kolk, B. (2014). *The Body Keeps the Score.* New York: Viking (p. 247).

6 van der Kolk, B. (2014). *The Body Keeps the Score.* New York: Viking (p. 247).

7 Wills, D. K. (2017). Healing Life's Trauma with Yoga. *Yoga Journal.* www.yogajournal.com/lifestyle/healing-lifes-traumas.

8 McLisky, A. (2023). Personal communication.

9 van der Kolk, B. (2014). *The Body Keeps the Score.* New York: Viking (p. 270).

10 Somerstein, L. (2010). Together in a Room to Alleviate Anxiety: Yoga Breathing and Psychotherapy. *Social and Behavioral Sciences, 5,* 267–71.

11 Bell, B. (n.d.). How Your Breath Affects Your Nervous System. *Feathered Pipe Ranch.* https://featheredpipe.com/feathered-pipe-blog/breath-affects.

12 Komori, T. (2018). The Relaxation Effect of Prolonged Expiratory Breathing. *Mental Illness, 10(1),* 6–7.

13 Desikachar, T.K.V. (1995). *The Heart of Yoga.* Rochester, VT: Inner Traditions International.

14 Pal, G., Agarwal, A., Karthik, S., Pal, P. & Nanda, N. (2014). Slow Yogic Breathing Through Right and Left Nostrils Influences Sympathovagal Balance, Heart Rate Variability, and Cardiovascular Risks in Young Adults. *North American Journal of Medical Sciences, 6(3),* 145–51.

15 Raghuraj, P., Ramakrishnan, A. G., Nagendra, H. R. & Telles S. (1998). Effect of Two Selected Yogic Breathing Techniques of Heartrate Variability. *Indian Journal of Physiology and Pharmacology, 42(4),* 467–72.

16 Srivastava, R. D., Jain, N. & Singhal, A. (2005). Influence of Alternate Nostril Breathing on Cardiorespiratory and Autonomic Functions in Healthy Young Adults. *Indian Journal of Physiology and Pharmacology, 49(4),* 475–83.

17 Kuppusamy, M., Kamaldeen, D., Pitani, R., Amaldas, J. & Shanmugam, P. (2017). Effects of Bhramari Pranayama on Health: A Systematic Review. *Journal of Traditional and Complementary Medicine, 8(1),* 11–16.

18 Kuppusamy, M., Kamaldeen, D., Pitani, R., Amaldas, J., *et al.* (2020). Effects of Yoga Breathing Practice on Heart Rate Variability in Healthy Adolescents: A Randomized Controlled Trial. *Integrative Medicine Research, 9,* 28–32.

19 Vashista, G. (2022). A Systematic Review of the Effects of Bhramari Pranayama on the Central and Autonomic Nervous System. Honours Dissertation, Auckland University of Technology, Tuwherea Open Repository. https://openrepository.aut.ac.nz/items/6cc20ad3-7881-414a-b733-0e7e03b1023e.

20 Garg, N. & Panda, S. K. (2021). Bhramari Pranayama: A Non-Pharmacological Approach Against Current Coronavirus Disease 19 Pandemic. *International Journal of Ayurveda and Pharma Research, 9(8),* 97–102.

21 Foster, D. (2016). Is Mindfulness Making Us Ill? *The Guardian.* www.theguardian.com/lifeandstyle/2016/jan/23/is-mindfulness-making-us-ill.

22 McGee M. (2008). Meditation and Psychiatry. *Psychiatry (Edgmont), 5(1)*, 28–41.

23 McGee M. (2008). Meditation and Psychiatry. *Psychiatry (Edgmont), 5(1)*, 28–41.

24 McGee M. (2008). Meditation and Psychiatry. *Psychiatry (Edgmont), 5(1)*, 28–41.

25 Gerritsen, R.J.S. & Band, G.P.H. (2018). Breath of Life: The Respiratory Vagal Stimulation Model of Contemplative Activity. *Frontiers in Human Neuroscience, 12*, 397.

26 de Manincor, M., Bensoussan, A., Smith, C., Fahey, P. & Bourchier, S. (2015). Establishing Key Components of Yoga Interventions for Reducing Depression and Anxiety, and Improving Well-being: A Delphi Method Study. *BMC Complementary and Alternative Medicine, 15*, 85.

27 de Manincor, M., Bensoussan, A., Smith, C., Fahey, P. & Bourchier, S. (2015). Establishing Key Components of Yoga Interventions for Reducing Depression and Anxiety, and Improving Well-being: A Delphi Method Study. *BMC Complementary and Alternative Medicine, 15*, 85.

28 Mason, H. & Gerbarg, P. (2018). Anxiety. In *Yoga for Mental Health*, ed. H. Mason & K. Birch. Pencaitland, Scotland: Handspring Publishing.

29 Mason, H. & Gerbarg, P. (2018). Anxiety. In *Yoga for Mental Health*, ed. H. Mason & K. Birch. Pencaitland, Scotland: Handspring Publishing.

30 Weintraub, A. (2004). *Yoga for Depression.* New York: Broadway Books.

31 Hanson, R. (2016). Yoga for Depression and Anxiety: A Systematic Review. *Master of Social Work Clinical Research Papers.* https://sophia.stkate.edu/msw_papers/590.

32 de Manincor, M., Bensoussan, A., Smith, C., Fahey, P. & Bourchier, S. (2015). Establishing Key Components of Yoga Interventions for Reducing Depression and Anxiety, and Improving Well-being: A Delphi Method Study. *BMC Complementary and Alternative Medicine, 15*, 85.

33 Tikle, Y. A. (2020). General Health Benefits of Pranayama W.S.R. to Effects on Respiratory System: An Ayurveda Review. *Journal of Drug Delivery and Therapeutics, 10(1)*, 215–17.

34 Weintraub, A. (2004). *Yoga for Depression.* New York: Broadway Books.

35 Raghuraj, P., Ramakrishnan, A. G., Nagendra, H. R. & Telles S. (1998). Effect of Two Selected Yogic Breathing Techniques of Heartrate Variability. *Indian Journal of Physiology and Pharmacology, 42(4)*, 467–72.

36 Brown, R. B. & Gerbard, P. L. (n.d.). *Yogic Breathing and Meditation: When the Thalamus Quiets the Cortex and Rouses the Limbic System.* www.semanticscholar.org/paper/Yogic-Breathing-and-Meditation-%3A-When-the-Thalamus-Brown-Gerbarg/b5d08de63dfaddfecfe7f29fffa159bd2017e193.

37 Weintraub, A. (2004). *Yoga for Depression.* New York: Broadway Books.

PILLAR SIX

1 Penman, S., Cohen, M., Stevens, P. & Jackson, S. (2012). Yoga in Australia: Results of a National Survey. *International Journal of Yoga, 5(2)*, 92–101.

Index